Sex in the Senior City

It Ain't Over,
It is Just An Old Game With New Rules

M. Maurice Abitbol, M.D.

SPUYTEN DUYVIL
New York City

ISBN 978-1-933132-56-3

Library of Congress Cataloging-in-Publication Data

Abitbol, M. Maurice.
Sex in the senior city / M. Maurice Abitbol.
p. ; cm.
Includes bibliographical references and index.
ISBN 978-1-933132-56-3 (alk. paper)
1. Older people--Sexual behavior I. Title.
[DNLM: 1. Sexual Behavior. 2. Aged.]
HQ30.A25 2007
306.7084'6--dc22

2007037002

Contents

WHY SEX IN THE SENIOR COMMUNITY?

The following two case histories introduce the problems faced by seniors about their sexuality.

I am now 77 years, a widower for the last five years after my wife died suddenly. Our family doctor said it was a cerebral hemorrhage. We have been sexually active all our life up to the time she died. I entered an assisted-living group home four years ago. Not that I was sick or anything, but I could not concentrate on things such as cooking, keeping my apartment clean, and so on. Frankly, I started having some lapse of memory that did not disturb me much but disturbed others. Like for instance, one day I walked out of the building to get the newspaper but I forgot to put my street clothes on and I was still wearing my pajamas. Anyway I like this institution very much and they take good care of you although I find it expensive.

I have a problem, however. There is a nice lady about my age and her apartment is two doors down across the hall. From the day I moved in, we recognized each other. We first talked to each other, then ate together and within a week or so, by mutual agreement, we had sex in her bedroom. At first the management of the place pretended to ignore us but when the guard making midnight rounds became aware that one of us was spending the night in the other's bedroom, they asked us to stop it. They did not want us to leave because they did not want to lose the money, neither did we want to leave because to live there was very convenient. Our worst enemy was the nursing supervisor, an old spinster, a bitch, who I think was simply jealous. I was told that our romance was not the first she interfered with and there were quite a few in the institution. She even notified our next of kin. My son found it amusing and so did one of her daughters, but her other daughter was rather embarrassed and asked her mother to be very discreet. We finally came to an understanding which was similar to the one of other couples in the same situation. As long as the nursing supervisor was on duty there was no expression of intimacy, just companionship. When she was off duty we became free. The other rule was that when the guard made rounds at midnight everybody should be in his or her room. This was not always practical because most of us in the place go to bed early. We managed anyway, because I get up frequently at night to go to the bathroom, and she has difficulty falling asleep until I join her. We have been like that for the last four years until a couple of months ago when the doctor of the place told me that she started showing early signs of Alzheimer's disease. I will stick with her as long as I can and I know that if it was not for my continuous attention to her and care for her, she would be required to leave the place because the institution is not equipped to handle this kind of disease. For the time being things are alright, to the relief of her two daughters who are horrified at the idea that they may have to take her back.

* * *

I am 72 years old, a retired bus driver, and I have been divorced since the age of 50. Our son was twenty years old at the time my wife and I divorced, and although he had some drug problems, he got out of it and is now happy with his own family. The main reason for our divorce was a sexual maladjustment. We both wanted to have sex, but it appeared that we never wanted it at the same time. She preferably wanted sex in the morning when I was in a rush to go to work, and I would have preferred it in the evening after supper before we went to sleep and she was not interested at that time. On weekends she always wanted to sleep late and I always got up early to go fishing. We had some marriage counseling but it did not do much. Besides a couple of years before the divorce I got involved with my wife's sister-in-law who just got divorced. Since then and until now I have been wandering from one sexual affair to another. For the last ten years I have been living with a lady, fifteen years younger than I am. I have been criticized all around about my sexual life: my son, my daughter-in-law who never wanted to meet my companion, my brother and sister and their spouses, and the priest from our church who kept telling me that I am and always have been living in sin. The lady I live with practically had to break up with all her family and friends after she moved in with me. I do not understand and I am really mad about this general condemnation, and I know many people of my age in this situation who cannot have a peaceful sexual life because of interference. We are not breaking the law, we are not harming anybody, and we like to be together. We do not want to get married because we both want to keep our freedom to terminate this relationship if one of us does not enjoy it anymore. Besides, I am suffering from high blood pressure and should I become incapacitated by a heart attack or cerebral hemorrhage, I would not want to become a burden to her. You have talked to many people of my age about their sexual life. Do you think I am doing something wrong?

Answer. Certainly not.

In *Sex and the City*, Samantha is the one who is most sexually active and the most diversified in the selection of her sexual partners. In one show, a rich, old gentleman, perhaps in his 70s, proposed a sexual affair to Samantha after supplying her with loads of jewelry. Once they were both naked in bed, the gentleman excused himself to go to the bathroom. As he got out of bed, Samantha had the opportunity to look at all his wrinkled skin, mostly his flabby hips. That turned her off immediately and she lost all sexual interest. While he was still in the bathroom, she quickly put on her clothes and walked out of his apartment, leaving all the jewelry behind. One can draw many conclusions from this scenario.

- Sex is the privilege of the young and healthy with firm skin and hips. Elderly are not fit for sex.
- It is 'sacrilegious' for young people to get sexually involved with old people. There is no price high enough to be paid by old people to have sex with young people.
- There is no senior way to have sex. There is only the young way. The only thing seniors can do is watch on TV or video cassette how the young perform sex, and try to imitate them.

The conclusion of this story is that *Sex and the City* describes sex as it is commonly conceived, i.e., only in the young and not in old people. To get an idea of a sexual life that includes old people, we have to go to *Sex in the Senior Community*. This is described in the following chapters.

Why a book on sexuality in senior citizens? The answer is very simple. When there were only a few seniors a century ago, their problems were minimal. Their problems were handled by their family, or completed ignored. No young adult who took his parent(s) to live with him or her was ever concerned about the parents' sexual needs. But now the general population is aging and the senior population is increasing. This raises multiple senior problems including the problem of senior sexuality. The same way it was embarrassing for the younger generation to talk about sex fifty years ago, the same way it is embarrassing to talk about senior sexuality today. Yet, it is now coming out slowly to the open, although still at the whispering stage. My first interviews provoked shock, anger, disbelief, repulsion and even rejection. Not anymore.

Senior citizens rarely expressed hostility to this investigation, at least not afterward. Many seniors complained that all they hear about their sexuality are jokes, ridiculous remarks, gossip, fantasies, distorted realities and most of all occasional scandals. They are aware of the reality of their sexuality which they would like studied, they would like it to be better known, and to have some qualified and knowledgeable person they could refer to for advice.

The main subject of conversation with senior citizens is of course their health. I learned that if I wanted to get a thorough sexual history I first had to patiently hear their whole medical history. Only when this was over, and it never really was over because they often kept coming back to it, then I could cautiously and thoroughly approach their complete sexual history. With patience and caution and through experience I had no problem getting their sexual history. In fact, I found out that senior citizens, mostly males but also females, very often talk between themselves about their sexual problems, and this is understandable because they have no one else to talk to. Many of them were delightfully surprised to find an attentive and qualified ear, something they said they never had before. Many seniors, I found, were occupied, if not preoccupied, with sex.

Mrs. Rosalind is a 67-year old divorcee, mother of three children, who came to see me for a gynecological evaluation because of a persistent vaginal irritation. She openly told me that she had masturbated at least twice a week since her divorce.

She went to see her regular gynecologist for this vaginal irritation and he performed the usual work-up including Pap smear and vaginal culture which all turned out to be negative. When she told him about her masturbation practice, he coldly told her to stop it and that would clear the irritation. She did not want to stop however and she understood that she was no longer welcome in her gynecologist's office because even the nurse receptionist who used to be friendly, but who must have read in her chart about her masturbation, had suddenly become cold. She changed gynecologist but the results were almost similar. She thought that this new gynecologist, who was rather young, would be more understanding. He was not. She was embarrassed and he even gave her the impression that he was repulsed with her masturbation. He told her that this was a practice for teenagers, that she should act her age and stop it immediately. She was rather annoyed with this medical attitude. She was harming nobody, she preferred masturbation rather than being exposed to all kinds of men whom she found more and more difficult to approach. She always had sexual urge and this was the only way to calm herself. Why did the doctors make her feel humiliated and abnormal?

I reassured her immediately that there was nothing abnormal with her masturbation and that it is a common practice among women who were desirous for sexual activity but lacked a sexual partner. I even stated that some married women combined masturbation with heterosexual activity in order to reach orgasm fully. On careful examination it was obvious that she presented a thinning of the vaginal mucosa, what is (wrongly) called 'senile vaginitis' and which responds easily to an estrogen ointment. I recommended that she use this medication as a lubricant during masturbation and apply it in the vagina at lease three times a week after her shower. I carefully went over her masturbation technique, recommended that she thoroughly wash her hands before masturbation, cut her nails short and always file them. Within two weeks of these suggestions and treatment her irritation cleared completely and she returned to her masturbation without any problems.

I noticed very quickly that non-cooperation came more from people involved in the care of the senior citizens than from the seniors themselves. Members of the family, religious ministers, administrators of nursing homes, managers of gated communities, medical personnel in charge of geriatrics, even security personnel, were all of the same opinion: there is no senior sexuality and, if there is any, it should not be talked about. This attitude reminded me of the shock expressed by the wife of the Archbishop of Canterbury when she heard of the theories of evolution as proposed by Charles Darwin: "We descend from the Apes! I hope it is not true, and if it is true, I hope it will never be known!" Well, senior sexuality is real and true and the purpose of this manuscript is to make it known. These people around seniors, often children of the seniors, have already made up their mind about the way of life of the seniors in practically every aspect including sexuality. It is unbelievable how much these surrounding people attempt to regulate the seniors' life, right down to the least detail. It seems to me that, having been under the order of their parents during their youth, the children now consider that it is their turn to educate their parents and boss them around. Currently, more and more seniors are attempting to liberate themselves in order to live an independent life whenever possible and to organize themselves in independent communities. Of course, when there is a physical or mental handicap, seniors depend on professional help. This does not always mean full control, but unfortunately this is how it often ends up.

The Danger of Ignoring Senior Sexuality

I am now 65 years old. When I finished high school at the age of 18 I went to work as a cashier in a department store. I had a few dates here and there. Then I started to go out seriously with the chief of my division who was 19 years older than I. I was 20 years old at the time and rather inexperienced in dating. He was the first man I had sex with. I did not mind the difference in age because I loved him, or at least I thought I did. I did not understand what he meant when he said that I should take precautions. At any rate, after a couple of months of this relationship I became pregnant. He was shocked because he thought I was using a diaphragm, something I had never heard of. There was no free abortion at that time and anyway the very idea of an abortion repulsed both of us. We were attached to each other and one month later we were married. I had my first baby normally. Five, then twelve years later, I had my second and third child. I would consider this a relatively happy marriage, although money was tight and there were some arguments here and there. I was frustrated after 20 years of marriage that we had sex less and less although discretely, then openly, I asked for it. But he was obese and had a touch of diabetes. When I reached the age of 45 (he was 64), he suddenly informed me that he could no longer have an erection and had to give up sex. I was devastated because at that time I was, if anything, more than ever desirous of sex. I had an early menopause and sex would not be inhibited by fear of pregnancy because I was never good at any form of birth control. We tried everything from specialists to regular medicine to quack medicine. Nothing worked and my husband never had an erection after that. I tried masturbation and all kinds of artificial penis and vibrator. The whole thing repulsed me and I ended up with vaginal irritations necessitating medical care. I was raised with high moral standards and any affair was out of the question, although there were frequent direct, and not so direct, propositions.

My husband died of severe diabetes at the age of 68, leaving me a widow at the age of 48. I was still beautiful, with a slim body, and highly desirous for sex. I would get orgasmic sex two to three times a week very easily. I tried an affair, but the man was brutal, asking for all kinds of bizarre and embarrassing sex such as anal intercourse, which was very painful. Besides he mostly wanted sex when he was drunk. I was embarrassed and even ashamed of the relationship and I ended it quickly. I never had any other sexual affair. I now sleep very poorly and wake up frequently in the middle of the night. I also have become irritable.

* * *

I am now 65 years old. Two of my three children are married; the oldest is now 45, a successful business man with children of his own; my second son is happily married and has a daughter; my third child is a 28 year old beautiful girl who is hoping to be married soon.

Q. Have you reconsidered marriage since you became a widow?

A. Yes, a few times, but my family needs me. I baby sit often, and I am always available to help in any occasion.

Q. How would your children feel if you were to remarry?

A. It depends. The oldest one would not like it because he needs my help with his large family. He and his wife appear to be selfish because they take me for granted on many occasions. They continually say I am a part of their family. My son keeps telling me that I am a second mother to his children and I imagine he would consider my remarrying an act of treason.

The wife of my second son is involved with her own mother who appears to be domineering. They all would rather keep me away from their family and my son would not care one way or another if I remarried.

My daughter would definitely like me to remarry. We lived together until last year when she moved to her own place. She does not want me to visit her apartment because she thinks I go through her rooms and closets to find out if a man is living there. In fact, one day we had a terrible argument and she suggested that I should remarry so that I would get off her back.

Q. Would you mind if your daughter lived with someone without getting married?

A. I would not like it, but I would adjust to it.

Q. So far you told me about your children's feelings if you remarry. How about your own feelings?

A. Well, my own feelings are determined by my children's feelings, especially the oldest who has taken some kind of responsibility for the entire family since his father's death. I would consider remarriage as some kind of betrayal to the memory of my husband and to my children. I am afraid they may feel I rejected them and that I would no longer want to have anything to do with them. If I were to remarry, it would have to be with their total approval.

Q. Since you are so desirous for sex and so full of sex appeal, would you consider living with somebody without getting married?

A. This would be out of the question. What would my children think of me? What would my daughters-in-law think of me? My daughter's fiancé would break off his engagement. I would have to stop my relationship with my whole family.

Q. Do you have sexual fantasies?

A. All the time. In fact, it is so frequent it reaches a level of obsession.

Q. Would you care to discuss these sexual fantasies?
A. No. It is too embarrassing. You would never guess the kind of sexual aberrations I have; I fantasize about sexual perversion and homosexuality.
Q. Do you have sexual dreams?
A. Often. The sexual activities in my dreams are more peaceful than my sexual fantasies. I often dream of one or two boyfriends I had as a teenager. I dream of kissing, hugging, petting, and sexual involvement.
Q. What would your reaction be if your learned that one of your children, your daughter for instance, was homosexual?
A. No chance, there is no homosexuality in my family.
Q. Is there any aspect of your current sexual attitude that we did not cover?
A. I would like to know if my current position (lack of sexual activity and sexual dreams and fantasies) is normal for a women my age?
Q. There is no standard of normality in your position. What you are is normal for you.

It is a well known psychological fact that when a problem is repressed, hidden, or worst of all ignored, the problem becomes explosive in nature. Under current conditions, it would be very helpful for the welfare of the senior community to talk openly about their sexuality and look deeply into it, the way we now talk openly about sexuality of younger people. The way similar studies have been helpful to younger generations, hopefully this study will be as helpful for seniors.

Currently, the senior community is very confused about sexuality. They are wondering if they are doing the wrong thing or not doing the right thing. They are concerned with what is 'normal' and what is not. They are obsessed with what everybody will think of them in this matter. They are afraid to appear ridiculous in their sexual desire, if any. Mostly they do not know what their sexuality should be and therefore refer to the sexual pattern of the younger generation as the model of performance; they refer to it constantly because they have no other model to refer to and worry about not being up to it. They constantly forget that the factors determining sexuality in the young are different from their own factors and therefore the two sexualities are different. This manuscript will attempt to bring all their questions into the open, in an attempt to find an answer to some of them at least. Mostly, the manuscript will not ignore a problem which cannot be ignored.

It is already a complex problem to delve into the sexuality of the adult population because of the implication of numerous factors such as biological drive, child bearing, intimacy, love, etc. These drives are natural and considered normal, whatever 'normal' means. But when we get to study sexuality in senior citizens, the problems are much more complex because the classic motivations are reshuffled: no more biological drive, no pregnancy or fear of it. Intimacy and/or love may or may not have been present before senior age and now may or may not still be present. In adult life, the man-woman relationship has more or less been traditionally consecrated: the man is outside at work and the woman is at home taking care of the house and children. This 'division' of work has priority over everything else and might even have played a role in keeping husband and wife together. This equilibrium, already shaken in our modern society, is further shaken for seniors because the children left the house and the man retired at home. How the senior man and the senior woman will relate is a completely different ball game.

I have interviewed young and middle age couples who express tremendous concern about aging because they feel once the children are gone and there is no more biological sex drive, they are afraid their relationship may disintegrate. On the contrary, I have also met couples who looked forward to senior life because all the children would be gone, there would be no more menstrual periods and fear of pregnancy, and they would have all the space and time for privacy and intimacy. Sexuality in old age is an open field. Its moral, social, and biological aspects have not been investigated much in a scientific and objective manner, away from prejudice and false pride.

Of all the plights and predicaments that seniors have to deal with, one of the most important is their sexuality because it is ignored, or not taken seriously, or met with hostility. The result is that seniors themselves are confused on the subject.

The great danger in looking at senior sexuality is to brush it off as a dirty subject or as non-existent. Love and sex have been and still are the greatest motivating forces in mankind, and there is no reason to deny this role in seniors. The greatest error that can be done in the present study is to look at it as some kind of pornographic investigation. In view of the reality of expanding old age, we will be depriving it of its vitality if we deprive or attempt to deprive it of its sexuality. Sexuality is a reality in old age, although possibly a different reality. Humans are creative by nature when they are in equilibrium and in perfect harmony with their mind, physical health, and emotions. Nothing disturbs this equilibrium and harmony more than a disturbed sexuality. To misjudge or to deny sexuality in old age (assuming it is there) is to interfere with the essence and meaning of life itself in old age. There is an increasing interest in studying the various aspects of life in the increasing senior citizenry, and this should include their sexual life. This trend should be encouraged, not inhibited. We will approach many unanswered questions:

Is there sex in senior citizens, and, if so, how much?
How does it vary with further aging?
How different is it from adult sex?
What motivates seniors in looking forward to or in avoiding sex?

The Meaning of Statistics

During the research part of my career I always concerned myself with the statistical significance of my work. Let us first define the meaning of statistics. It means to study a problem in a representative segment of a population and attempt to apply the conclusions drawn from that small segment to the whole population.

Ideally, of course, it would be very accurate to study all the individuals from the whole population. This is usually impossible because the whole population is too large. This is also unnecessary because if one carefully selects a segment of the whole population that is as accurately as possible representative of the whole population, the result from the representative segment are similar and can be safely extended to the whole population. Therefore, the problem in statistics is how much the small segment that is selected for investigation is representative of the whole population. Too often, unfortunately, the studied segment is not representative of the whole population. This is the reason why two or more scientists who study a similar phenomenon end up with different conclusions, because the representative segment was selected differently. I have seen many researchers take the easy way out in selecting a representation. Careful representation is very expensive and requires a tremendous effort. Researchers often look for the easiest representation they can reach. More and more researchers no longer mention the size of the basic population from which they extract their representation. They just keep increasing the representation to a higher number in order to impress their audience. They do not mention how the representation is selected. They are concerned mostly with a high representative number and therefore they are more biased. Let me now take a few concrete examples of misrepresentation that I find significant.

In order to avoid misrepresentation, some researchers extend as much as possible the representative segment. For instance, instead of studying 50 subjects out of 1000 population (or 5%) they study 100 subjects out of the same 1000 population (10%). If the representative segment is increased from 50 to 100 out of the same 1000 population, the value of the statistic increases. But, if the representative segment is increased from 50 to 100 and at the same time the population is increased from 1000 to 2000, the value of the statistics is scarcely increased, still 5%. Let us take an example. A researcher wants to study the value of Vitamin C intake in preventing flu during the winter. He selects 50 children out of a total of 1000 children in a school. But he made an error: the 50 children belong to the highest income family because they are the easiest to approach. The correct way to avoid this error would be to increase his representative segment from 50 to 100 children by including children of families with low income within the same school of 1000 pupils, because another researcher studying only 50 children from low income families would draw different conclusions. Instead he increased his representation by including 50 children also of high income families from another school with 1000 children also. He doubled his representation, but also doubled the basic population with the same error. In spite of an increase in representation, he did not increase the value of his statistics. Now the same biased study can be extended to 100 schools with a total basic population of 100,000 children and a representation of 5000 children. The researcher impressed his audience with the high number of 5000 subjects. Yet, he took the easy way out when selecting his representation. His study would have been of much more value if it was limited to 1000 children in a school of 1000 children from an average neighborhood. He would have had only 1000 cases to present instead of 5000, but the results would have had much more significance. A general audience would not be impressed, but qualified statisticians would be. This mistake is made all the time by researchers who think they can diminish the misrepresentation by increasing the size of the selected segment **and** at the same time increasing the total population.

Another scientific technique to reach higher results is the double-blind method. For example, 100 children are given Vitamin C pills and 100 other children placebo pills that look and taste like Vitamin C pills. The two categories of children are chosen randomly, then compared. With this method, one does not need many subjects to reach accuracy.

During my college years I was interested in hypnosis. I found it fascinating that a stage hypnotist could randomly pick a person from the audience and put him/her in a state of deep hypnosis. I joined a school of hypnosis, which I attended three evenings a week for four months, and then I graduated. I performed poorly however and I could barely hypnotize anyone. I was desperate. Then I started to attend the performance of a famous stage hypnotist whom I had become friendly with during my attendance at the school for hypnosis. After a while he initiated me into all the tricks of the trade. "Your skill, he explained to me, is not so much in the technique of hypnosis, which is rather easy to learn and which you skillfully possess, but in learning to recognize a subject receptive to hypnosis, what we call a good medium. They are few and far apart but you can always find a couple in a general audience of at least 100 people. Suppose I am on stage in front of an audience of say 100 persons. I ask the audience for volunteers to be hypnotized. I know by experience that good mediums for hypnosis always volunteer and that if there is a good medium in the audience, he/she will be among the volunteers. I usually get 7-8 volunteers on the stage. I observe them carefully starting some hypnosis techniques and right away I pick out a couple of them as excellent mediums. I find some excuse to send the others back to their seats and I work on the two or three selected ones. I immediately recognize the most suitable among them because he/she is already half hypnotized. I perform my amazing show on the one I selected from an audience of 100 subjects. I repeat this performance two to three times a week. I sometimes go to a party of fifteen to twenty persons. All I have to do is say I am a hypnotist (sometimes people at the party have already heard of me) and immediately the good mediums gravitate around me. I recognize the best medium for a show. If I do not recognize a receptive subject, I always find an excuse for not performing. Now I have to be honest with you and confess that I have a few excellent mediums for hypnosis that are on my payroll or who are glad to be repeat volunteers and I often arrange for one or two of them to be in the audience when I run out of good mediums." Let us now analyze statistically this hypnosis performance. To the average layman this stage hypnotist is a magician. He can hypnotize anybody, anywhere. He hypnotized thousands of people, and I believe it. The other side of the story is that he hypnotized only one percent of the audience he was exposed to, and this one percent is not representative of the general audience he was exposed to. People forget that 99 percent of the people he was exposed to were not and could not be hypnotized by him or by anybody else for that matter. His representative segment of the population is a biased representation, because they were highly selected. If the candidates for stage hypnosis had been selected haphazardly by some other person, he would have failed miserably. He hides this misrepresentation by increasing the representative segment ("I hypnotized 2,000 people"), forgetting to mention that this high number is biased, selected from a population of maybe 200,000. I am still not a good hypnotist but I conducted a few good shows during my lifetime and, as an obstetrician, I delivered a few patients, very few, under hypnosis without any sedation or anesthesia.

Let me give another significant example concerning the performance of the average soldier in the American Armed Forces. During the Vietnam War, G.I.'s were drafted by the Selective Service System, and the individuals in the Armed Forces were more or less representative of the young male population of that time, although there were some volunteers. At any rate, the war was not popular and hardly anyone wanted to go to the battle front. Recruitment for the subsequent wars (Gulf War, Kosovo, Afghanistan) was completely different. They were all volunteers or from the National Reserves, which were also volunteers. They were ready to kill the enemy and ready to die. Even from this first layer of volunteers, individuals were chosen who were highly advanced in the sophisticated technology of modern warfare. They were very disciplined and would not spread rumors about what is going on at the battle front. In no way could these modern soldiers be considered representative of their generation, the way the soldiers in the Vietnam War were. The former represent a highly selected segment not representative of their generation, while the later are. The performance of the two types of soldiers is completely different and it would be a mistake to confuse both. It would be a mistake to categorize the qualifications of the modern soldier, then generalize and extend them to a general draft. I do not want to delve into politics, but I hope I showed one small reason why the Vietnam war was a disaster and the subsequent wars were a success.

Although coming from different fields, the above examples will help us evaluate and criticize statistical reports on the study of human sexuality, namely by Kinsey, Pomeroy and Martin in 1948. It was the first extensive report on a subject that was considered 'off limits' previously. This study had a tremendous impact on our society because it was conducted in a scientific and objective manner. Criticisms have piled up since however, which in no way tarnish its value. I hope my manuscript on the study of senior sexuality will also have an impact, the way the Kinsey et al. report had on sexuality in the young and adult. In this endeavor, I would like to avoid statistical errors made by Kinsey et al., and similarly by other authors. Their representative population is tremendous, the largest one on the subject. Their series involved subjects by the tens of thousands. But they fell into the usual trap of thinking it is enough to present a very large series in order to have statistical value. My criticisms are multiple.

These authors never mentioned the size of the basic population from which their subjects came. When they studied 100 volunteer inmates in jail, did they provide the size of the population in jail? When they reported on 20 volunteer prostitutes, we do not know what the prostitute population was in that neighborhood. It was only in the college population that they were more or less accurate, although they did not mention how many colleges were unsuccessfully approached for their study. Of the 12,000 reported cases, only 26% were from total population; 74% were volunteers, i.e., partial population. The results from the total groups were different from the partial volunteer group. Even in the total groups, they reported only on benign elements such as masturbation or nocturnal emissions and not on serious elements such as homo or heterosexuality.

Besides, how can they mix a total college population with a limited non-college representation? Yet, they present the results as coming from a general population. Besides, they studied college students at a time when colleges were in a state of turmoil; therefore this was a limited and even biased representation of a general population. College students may be the front runners of many things, including sexuality, but they never have been representative of society as a whole in sexuality or in any other field for that matter. At any rate, excessive sexuality that we attributed to college students a generation ago at the time of the Kinsey report, has more or less subsided and currently they are not much different sexwise from the rest of society.

My criticism is serious because the authors mentioned that most subjects were volunteers. This is a dangerous concept, although it is very commonly practiced. If they study only volunteers it means that they did not study non-volunteers. It means that we have no idea about the sexual behavior of the non-volunteer population. The reasons people do and do not volunteer indicate two different types of populations with opposite or at least different sexual profiles. This reminds us of the volunteers for the study of Vitamin C, of hypnosis, or of Armed Forces where the selected volunteers were arbitrarily made representative of the whole population. There are ample reasons to extend this criticism to the Kinsey report, which reported only on volunteers. To extend the conclusions of the volunteer population to the non-volunteer population is biased and scientifically unsound. Kinsey et al. are to be praised for their large series of 10,000. From a scientific point of view however it would have been more accurate to study all the students of only one college and report on the reasons given by those students who refused to participate. It might not have been more spectacular but it would be more sound and more accurate from the scientific point of view.

During my scientific career, I always have been suspicious of very large series, especially when the size of the basic population is not listed, and when all subjects are volunteers. In our study on senior sexuality we will report on the extent of the basic population in an attempt to reach most, if not all of it. We will register the refusal of those who do not want to participate and the reason for their refusal. We stayed away from volunteers picked at random from a general population group. For instance, when we approached a retirement home, we never limited ourselves to volunteers, but attempted to get a response or a lack of response from the whole population in that group and our intention was not limited to reaching only volunteers for interviews but the total community. Some examples will explain how we reached that goal.

Questionnaire Proposed to Seniors

N.B. Please do not mention your name, address, phone number, or any information that may lead to your identification.

A. General Questions:

Sex - Age - Race - Religion and how much involved
Profession and date of retirement, if retired
Economical level
Education: Elementary, High School, College, Post-College
Alcohol, Smoking
Hobbies in retirement, if retired
Physical exercise
Current health status

B. Marital History:

a) 1st marriage, from what age to what age
b) 2nd marriage, from what age to what age
c) Currently widower, widow, divorced
d) Living with a partner, not married, or living alone

C. Sex Life Prior to Age 55:

Males: Frequency of sexual activity: how many times a week or month
Any experience and/or expertise for inducing climax in sexual partner

Females: Frequency of sexual activity, how many times a week or month. Percentage of orgasms
Preparation by partner for sexual climax

Any extra-marital activity in married couples or for seniors living with a companion

Masturbation: Isolated, prior to, or after heterosexual sex

Homosexuality

D. Sex Life After Age 55: divided in 5-year period up to present age

Frequency of Sexual Activity (since age 55 to present):
List approximate frequency for each period
1w, 2w, 3w, etc. means weekly frequency
1m, 2m, 3m, etc. means monthly frequency
1y, 2y, 3y, etc. means yearly frequency

Example for age 72:

55-60	60-65	65-70	70-75	75-80	80-85	85-90	90-95	95-100	100+
3W	2M	4Y	4Y	N/A	N/A	N/A	N/A	N/A	N/A

E. The Sexual Act

Initiation:
Does the male make the first approach when desirous of sex
Does the female make the first approach

Women: Willing, looking forward to
Consenting, i.e., not planned but do not refuse
Only under pressure after numerous requests
Refuse

Men: Initiating
Not initiating

Modes of Approach:

1. General body contact including kissing, either naked or partially clothed
2. No preparation: direct penetration by erect penis
3. One partner prepares the other:
a. female: penis manipulation, mouth-penis
b. male: breasts, clitoris, vaginal, mouth-clitoris
4. Both at the same time prepare each other

Protection Against V.D.

Male or female condom

Penetration:

Gentle, lubricant
Brutal, painful
Vaginal narrowing

Sexual Position:

Male above
Female above
Side position, facing each other or male facing back of female
Sitting
Vaginal penetration from the back
Anal intercourse
More than one position from above list

Duration of Act:

Time interval between two thrusts (slow, rapid)

Number of thrusts before orgasm

Orgasm:
For women: Definition of it: number of vaginal spasms; general contraction, then relaxation
Satisfaction in partner's orgasm
Indifference to orgasm and/or lack of it
Frustration for not reaching it and repressed or silent anger

For men: How easily reached
Anxiety in reaching it
Frustrated for not reaching it
Frustration when female partner does not reach orgasm

Who reaches first and does the other wait?

Post Coitus:
Isolation feeling
Turning back, falling asleep, walking away
Continues hugging
Ecstasy

F. Additional Questions

Availability of Sex Partners:
Marital
Extra-marital
Prostitute
Desirous but no partners (mostly women)
No desire

Masturbation:
Male
Female (finger, vibrator, other objects)
Isolated or combined with heterosexuality

Homosexuality:
Regular homosexual partner
Casual partner
Combined or not combined with heterosexuality

Sexual orientation :
a. Heterosexual
b. Homosexual
c. Bisexual

If you have had more than one sexual orientation in your life, please give your approximate age for each sexual orientation:

Heterosexual: age ______to______
Homosexual: age ___ to _____
Bisexual: age ___ to _____

Examples:
a. heterosexual: age 17 to present
b. homosexual: 21 to 51
c. bisexual: none

Methods of Approach and Anonymity

I am a 71 year old widow. My husband passed away five years ago. He was a heavy smoker and he had lung cancer. I have two daughters, one a school teacher married to the principal of the school where she works, another married to a priest. I have five grandchildren and it is a delight to have the whole family together in my home a few times a year. I am embarrassed to say it but for the last two years I am having an affair with a gentleman a couple of years younger than I am. He is not living with his wife anymore but they are not divorced, at least this is what he says. Nobody, absolutely nobody, knows anything about this. He comes once or twice a week to my house supposedly to fix anything or to do the gardening and he enters the house through the back door. Or I meet him in the parking lot of the supermarket where he picks me up in his car and we go to his house, enter the garage, then he closes the garage door before I get out of his car. We enjoy each other's company tremendously, sexual and otherwise. We would like to go on some vacation cruise, but I am afraid of the gossip. If my affair becomes known, it will disturb the reputation of my children's families.

Q. Did you even think of discussing it openly with one of your daughters?

A. No. I know that my daughter, the priest's wife, came to see you and asked you about the questions you are asking me about sex in seniors. I also know that she exploded in indignation when you asked her opinion about any sexual activity on my part. First, I did not want this interview at all. The reason I agreed is to make sure that whatever I told you about my private life would never be known or suspected by my children or children-in-law, or anybody else.

Q. I assure you that in no way will it ever be known. All information you give me is purely confidential, and anyway all the documents are destroyed after they have been tabulated and analyzed. Do you think that your secret life will ever be known by your daughters or do you think that they suspect that you are involved with your companion?
A. I am not sure. Sometimes I feel angry. What am I afraid of? Why do I have to account to anybody for my behavior? I have a friend of mine who is in a position similar to mine, except that her companion is fully accepted by her children. Why don't I have the same luck? Sometimes I am concerned that the secrecy surrounding my relationship is so excessive that it might ruin it.

A plan was made to investigate all the subjects above 55 in a specific community, a gated community for instance. We prepared with the cooperation of some members of that community who had heard of our investigation or who had been approached to arrange for such an investigation. These initial members promised their full cooperation in attempting to reach the **whole** community. The first step was to approach the Board of that community to proceed with the plan. The list, exact address and phone number of each member living in that community were secured, and a letter was sent to all of them explaining the purpose of the investigation and asking them to cooperate and attend seminars explaining what it is about. Two to three seminars at different days of the week and different hours of the day were arranged in an attempt to reach most of them. Absolute anonymity was promised that no mode of identification would be kept. We received phone calls from those who wanted to be interviewed. A questionnaire was presented to each member and a personal interview followed the return of the questionnaire. All questions regarding the questionnaire were answered and absolute anonymity was again guaranteed. All questionnaires and the list of community members were destroyed after all the data were tabulated. Interviews were conducted privately between the seniors and a social worker, usually a professional social worker or some trained volunteer. Married couples or people living together were interviewed separately.

The next step was a second letter sent to those members of that specific community who had not responded, proposing attendance at a personal seminar and/or a private visit to their home for the interview. In this second letter a telephone interview was proposed if the senior wished. Additional seniors were reached this way.

The third and last attempt was a phone call and sometimes a personal approach in an attempt to determine the cause for refusing the interview. This third group was divided into the following categories:

1. Could not be reached
2. Physically or mentally handicapped and could not talk
3. Refused any discussion and hung up
4. Refused to be interviewed and gave reason for refusal
5. Could not be categorized

As we became more experienced, this fifth category diminished as we managed, indirectly and through a third party, to find out the reason for non-interview.

One way or another, we managed to find out some answers for everybody in the community including those with no answers. We found out very quickly that had we limited ourselves only to those who volunteered and had we not attempted to reach the rest of the community, the statistical conclusions would have been much different. For instance, those who volunteered right away were mostly in the younger group and had an active sexual life, while those who did not volunteer were usually older and with limited sexuality. This will be detailed in the following statistical tables.

Another category of seniors was drawn from the medical practice of busy gynecologists, urologists, and specialists in general medicine. Here, too, we specified that the study would have value only if a specific group could be totally approached with an answer from each member of the group, with an explanation for those who were not interviewed, and for those without an explanation for refusing to participate, the percentage they represent within the group. Usually the secretary-receptionist handed a brochure to all the private patients explaining the purpose of the study. She made a list of all the patients 55 and older that were seen in the office for a specific period, for example, say a one-year period. She handed them a brochure, or more directly proposed an interview, or suggested attendance at a seminar that would explain the purpose of the study. The secretary-receptionist made a gentle approach either personally or by phone to those who had not responded within a month, proposing a home interview, a simple questionnaire without identification, a telephone interview, or their reason for refusal to be interviewed. The secretary-receptionist also kept a tabulation of those who refused to discuss the matter of the study.

Finally, a group of patients from the outpatient department, who were 55 years or older, were registered during a specific period. These patients were registered for a two-year period and were approached in a method similar to the previous group, getting from them either an interview or a questionnaire, or a refusal and the reason for it, or refusal with no reason, or could not be reached. Tabulations were kept of the different categories.

Whenever one is involved with a study concerning human sexuality, one quickly learns a basic rule, namely that the subject interviewed wants to remain anonymous. Some give the appearance of "I don't care" but most, if not all, of them like to remain anonymous in at least some details of their sexual profile. This rule is reinforced and becomes even more absolute when it applies to senior citizens. In this matter, seniors feel inhibited, fearful of being ridiculous or not normal, and are very reluctant to open up at least in the beginning. Senior citizens are basically eager to discuss their sexuality and learn about the general consensus of their age group. But they are adamant about not being identified. We never asked or recorded names and addresses. It was specifically stated that the sheet recording the data did not contain any identification data and when the sheet was given by social workers and secretaries for analysis, there was absolutely no way to identify the subjects who were interviewed. Whenever we interviewed a specific senior community, the word quickly spread that the study was completely anonymous and this encouraged the seniors to participate in the investigation.

All interviews were private as we never conducted group interviews, not even couples living together. Seminars helped only in terms of explaining the purpose and mechanism of the study and to strongly stress the absolute anonymity even between husband and wife or a couple living together. Some seniors learned that some other seniors had been interviewed, but they learned it from each other and not from us. We never discussed with the seniors the details of someone else's interview, not even husband and wife. We guaranteed that the personnel performing the statistical analysis had no way of identifying the name and address of seniors, and that all the reports would be destroyed after analysis. For the published interviews, any detail that could lead to identification was sufficiently or slightly altered so that identification became impossible. It was by reinforcing this absolute anonymity that we got many interviews and at least some answers, even a negative answer, from everybody so that we were able to tabulate each whole community.

Practically all the interviewed seniors were eager for the interviewer's opinion about their own sexuality or lack thereof, how they compared to others, and/or brought specific problems for advice and treatment. We never made any comment in this matter. All we did was to reassure each and every senior that their behavior was normal for them and there was never anything to be ashamed or guilty of, or embarrassed about. It was unbelievable how the seniors felt reassured when told that their sexual behavior, or lack of it, was perfectly normal and within normal expectations regardless what this behavior was or whether it was considered normal or abnormal. Many of them were torn between guilt in doing whatever they were doing or developed an aggressive tendency because they thought they were forbidden from doing what they would like to do. Constant reassurance that their behavior and their feelings were normal contributed to deeper 'confessions' and in bringing more and more people for interviews as they frequently talked to each other. Many seniors live a withdrawn and secluded life and the opportunity to open up to the attentive ear of the interviewer was welcomed.

There are some general comments concerning our interviews. We watched for exaggeration and paranoia, mostly in males. I recognized a couple of individuals with early Alzheimer's disease, early dementia, and Parkinson's. We watched for seniors with poor memory for recent events (early Alzheimer's disease) but sometimes very detailed memory of past events. We compared reports of spouses or living partners for accuracy, whenever possible.

General Analysis of the Approached Population

The last census of the population in the USA was carried in 1996, and 272.6 million people were registered (Table 1). There were 133.2 million males and 139.4 million females. The two sexes are more or less equal in number up to the age of 55, with slightly more males in early adulthood and slightly more women in late adulthood. However, beginning at age 55, the percentage of women in relation to men starts to increase, slowly at first, then more and more rapidly with advancing age. As of 55 years of age, there are ten percent more women than men, and after 85 there are twice as many women than men. In 1996, the U.S. population above 55 years of age was 54.8 million, of which 43.8% were males and 56.2% were female.

Table 2 shows how life expectancy has progressed and rapidly increased during the last century. In the beginning of the 20th century, the average life span was 48 years for women and 46 for men. Today, the average woman reaches 80 and the average man reaches 77. We will study later on the reasons and the consequences of this increased life span.

Our studied population was composed of 3396 individuals that were above 55 years of age: 1526 subjects or 44.9% were males, and 1870 subjects or 55.1% were females (Table 3). Our population, as far as repartition between the two sexes, is representative of the general U.S. population (Table 4). Table 4 shows the distribution by age of the U.S. population beyond 55 years of age, and Table 3 shows the distribution by age of the population that was approached in this study. These data are also presented in Figures 1 and 2. These tables and figures show that, within minimal variations, the repartition by age in our representative population is similar to the repartition by age of the population of the U.S. in general. Consequently, as far as age distribution is concerned the population that was approached in this study is representative of the whole population.

Of the 3396 seniors that have been approached (Table 5) for this study, 2722 or 80.2% were successfully interviewed. The other 674 seniors, or 19.8% either refused or had incomplete interviews (267 cases, or 7.8%) or were mentally handicapped (200 cases or 5.9%) or physically handicapped (207 or 6.1%). We have no idea about how many seniors among the general population would have had an incomplete interview or would have refused interview, but the relatively modest figure in our representative population (267 subjects or 7.8%) does not appear unreasonable and could relatively be safely extended to the whole population. As far as mental and physical handicaps (200 subjects or 5.9% and 207 subjects or 6.1% respectively), these figures are corroborated by the statistics for the U.S. Department of Health and other reliable sources and are therefore representative of the general population.

Table 6 shows the repartition by race and Table 7 shows the religious background. Again, these figures correspond to those of the general U.S. population. Table 8 shows the background of our representative population: some lived in relatively wealthy gated communities, others in assisted living of varying degrees, others were in a nursing home, and still others lived either alone or with relatives. Many came from the practice of private physicians, others were hospital clinic patients. All our patients were more or less evenly distributed among these different seniors. The conclusion, therefore, was that we could safely extend the conclusions that would be drawn from this study to the general senior population of the U.S.

Our representative population had a mode of living not different from the general population of the same age. They were married or single, living alone or with a family, or in a community or a nursing home. Their mode of living did not appear different from the general senior population (Table 9).

We certainly could have extended our representative population far beyond the 3396 cases that we had reached. We did not think this was indicated for many reasons. First and most important, once we reached this figure, the findings were more or less repetitive, and we did not think that we were learning anything new. We were more interested in a complete history and in reaching a whole community, than in extending our representation. Our goal was to reach accurate data and not so much extend data beyond limits. Besides, our impression and conclusion is that 3396 is a highly representative figure and we do not know of any similar study on senior sexuality that is nearly as extensive as ours. Not that we want to impress anybody by this high figure.

Table 10 is the basic table that will be constantly referred to during this investigation. It shows that, of the 3396 seniors that were approached, 2722 were satisfactorily interviewed for statistical analysis. Table 10 also shows repartition of the interviewed population by gender and by age.

While interviewing or attempting to interview our 3396 senior citizens, we became exposed to some of their relatives. Most of the time these were their children, but also other relatives such as siblings, distant relatives, or just close friends. We even interviewed three parents of our senior population. These relatives were casually encountered while we were attempting to approach the seniors, but some of them approached us directly because they wanted to know about our research project. Some were just curious, others were interested, but a few were hostile to the project. We did our best to explain the nature of the project, stressing strongly the complete anonymity and that there was no way to identify the interviewed subjects or their location. Most of those who were hesitant or hostile were reassured. We managed to approach 1502 adults, of which 569 were males, and 933 were females. We took this opportunity to ask them a few general questions such as:

1. What they think of seniors who are still married or even no longer married and how they are involved in sexual activity.
2. What they (the relatives) think their own sexuality will or should be when they grow older.

In summary we approached 3396 seniors and 1502 adults for the purpose of investigating senior sexuality. These series are by far the largest reported in the literature. Even Kinsey et. al. reported only on a couple of hundred seniors and even these subjects belonged to the youngest group of seniors.

Why Was 55 Chosen as the End of Adult Age and the Beginning of Senior Age

I am 71 years old. My husband is the same age. He was a car mechanic, and managed a car repair shop and gas station which he owned. I helped with the bookkeeping. It was a hard life because I had to raise a family of four children with the help of my widowed mother-in-law with whom I got along very well. We all lived above the repair shop. Our life was hectic between the home and the business. Our sexual life during those working years was haphazard and very irregular. My husband had his sexual requests at the oddest hours and only when the kids were at school and when my mother-in-law was shopping, or in the middle of the night when we thought everyone was sleeping. The most tense moment of our sexual life was one time late at night when in the middle of our sexual activity we found our daughter, then five years old, standing by our bed. She could not sleep and wanted a glass of water. We gave her the glass of water, put her to sleep between the both of us and forgot everything else. We never locked our bedroom and always told the children to come to our bedroom and wake us up if there was any problem. We were scared of a fire in view of the gas station below.

I always enjoyed sex and easily reached orgasm because my husband was very good at it. Orgasm, however, was reached infrequently for many reasons; fear of the children hearing us because my husband was very noisy during his orgasm and would easily wake up the children; fear of my mother-in-law hearing us from her bedroom which was just above ours; fear mostly of getting pregnant because I was bad at birth control and my husband would not hear of using a condom. My four pregnancies were not planned. There was also menstrual bleeding lasting ten days a month because I was suffering from uterine fibroids. This was corrected however at the age of 45 after I had a hysterectomy. We had a good time only a few days a year when we left the children with my mother-in-law and took a cruise.

Now everything has changed. My mother-in-law passed away about the same time as the last child left home. We worked so hard for more than thirty years and we decided to take an early retirement at the age of 56. We sold the business with a good profit, and we moved south to a lovely little home near the beach. No more worries about business, about the children, about noise waking up my mother-in-law, about the gas station burning, about getting pregnant, or about menses preventing sex. Both my husband and I are on our second honeymoon (or rather, our first real one) for the last fifteen years. We were having sex every second to third day and to this day we maintain the same frequency. I almost always reach orgasm because my husband is loving and very patient. Besides, we freely tell each other our desires and I do not hesitate to tell him where and how I can reach orgasm. We tell each other when one of us is desirous of sex. Besides, we do not have to tell each other anything as we quickly sense each other's sexual needs. We are very open about how and where we should touch each other, what position we should take, and so on. The only interference in our sex life is when one of us is sick. He also occasionally suffers from backache but we always find the proper position to get around that.

Q. Do you keep your pajamas on during sex?

A. No; we prefer to be naked, but occasionally one of us keeps the pajama on. In fact, when one of us is naked or one of us has pajamas on, it is a signal to the other about desire or lack of desire for sex.

Q. How do you feel about your bodies, sexually speaking.

A. My husband is very muscular and I have managed to keep my body in shape in spite of my pregnancies. I love his body physically and he always compares my body to an ancient Greek statue. Besides, we attend a physical education center to keep our bodies in shape. I also do frequent massage therapy. Of course, I started having wrinkles on my face and we jokingly talk about a face lift if we could get a reduced price for the two of us.

Q. How long do you think this active sex life will continue?

A. Forever. My mother told me one day that at the age of eighty, she and my father occasionally had sexual relations. I intend to beat her at it, if my husband and I stay alive.

Q. Is the sexual attraction of your bodies the only thing that keeps you together.

A. Not at all. There is a spiritual attraction that has developed between us during the last few years. We have common and separate interests that we both respect. We both like bridge and joined a bridge club. We both attend lectures on mysticism and are being educated about it. But I like sewing and attend a sewing group twice a week. He now likes sailing and he and some neighbors purchased a sailing boat. I am always afraid of an accident at sea, but he likes to go sailing the whole day, once or twice a week and I never object to it.

Q. If your husband dies first, would you consider sex with a new husband or a sexual companion?

A. No, I do not think so. I will always have him in mind and that would interfere in a sexual involvement with another partner. His memory will be enough for me to go on by myself.

Q. If you die first, would your husband look for another sexual partner?

A. I don't think so. But he enjoys sex so much, so I do not know. He will be free to do what he wants.

Q. Now that you've passed the age of bearing children, what is the function of sex in your life?

A. We never had sex in order to get pregnant. In fact, the fear of pregnancy interfered with and sometimes inhibited our sex life. I consider sex a mode of creating and/or reinforcing intimacy and love. Even if sexual activity is diminished or even suppressed, the love and intimacy persists. I am sure that if for some reason our sexual life is interrupted, our relationship will not be interfered with in any way.

Q. Is there any sexual position or any way to have sex, that you prefer?

A. We like them all and practice them all. However, I do not like oral or anal sex, although my husband would like that.

Q. Do you let him have his way in that matter?

A. Yes, but not frequently. He understands my objections.

Q. Are your friends aware in any way of the quality in your relationship?

A. Oh, yes. These kind of things you do not hide. Most of our friends know that we are very close and that our personal life is very intimate.

Q. Do you see sex movies?

A. A few times in the past. We are not interested.

Q. Do you have sexual fantasies?

A. No, I have only sexual realities.

Q. Any sexual dreams?

A. Occasionally; mostly pleasant dreams.

Q. Has one of you ever been unfaithful to the other?

A. Not me. I am sure not him either, although he has always been attractive and there were plenty of opportunities around.

Q. Do you have any questions?

A. Yes. Do you think I am a nymphomaniac?

My answer: No, madam, you are not. You are the sexual symbol for senior citizens of the future.

Many qualified people I discussed this study with wondered why I did not select 65 as the beginning of senior age, since this is the age considered today for retirement. I have many reasons for selecting the age 55 as the beginning of senior sexuality.

To begin with I never consider any age to be an age of retirement whether it is from activity in general or as we will see later, from sexual activity. The age at which people retire, whatever that word means, has tremendously varied in history. I imagine that before human society became organized, at the age of the Cave Man, practically nobody reached the age of forty. Men died at war or hunting; women died in childbirth and everybody died of infections and malnutrition. Up to a century ago, in spite of general social progress, in spite of agriculture, cattle raising, and industry, the average life span did not go beyond the mid forties. Today at the beginning of the third millennium, with progress in each and every field, the average person, if they take care of themselves and take advantage of all progress, can easily reach eighty and beyond. I will show later that there is a remarkable relationship between health and sexual activity. The point I am trying to make is that the age of retirement, which is variable in space and time, has nothing to do with sexual activity.

Rather, I consider the beginning of senior sexuality as the age in which the outlook, the purpose, and the motivations for sex have radically changed. Throughout this manuscript we will oppose sexuality of the young and adults to the sexuality of seniors. This will be summarized in further tables which will be discussed later on. The transition from the adult to the senior type of sexuality can be slowly progressive, or it may occur suddenly. However, my observations on the subject of human sexuality that have been going on over many decades led me to the conclusion that this transition occurs around 55 years of age. At that time menstruation and hormonal activity has disappeared in women. For men, this is the age where attraction to women has markedly slowed down or at least changed and this is the age where men have settled down in life: they have not retired yet, but either they slow down and start planning for retirement, or, at least, they stop planning ambitious goals and consider themselves settled. If there is a tendency to be a playboy, it stops at around 55. Sexual search slows down. Of course these are general remarks with multiple exceptions, but my final impression is that at 55, one important transition towards a new life, specifically sexual life, is occurring. These are the reasons I consider 55 as the age of transition from adult to senior sexuality.

The main transition is that before 55, the family life was important. After 55, care of the family is terminated and most of the time children are either gone or have outside activities that do not require parents' interference and/or guidance. Before 55, sex was done in relation to pregnancy, either how to get pregnant or how to avoid it. After 55, pregnancy is completely out of the mind of the sex partners and, as we will see later, there is a complete reevaluation as to what does or does not motivate sexual activity.

What Adults Think Their Sexuality Will Be When They Become Seniors

This is illustrated in the following two case histories representing two opposite points of view.

I am forty years old, mother of five children from four to sixteen years of age. I came to visit my seventy year old father who is in a nursing home. I became pregnant with my first child as soon as I got married. My husband barely makes enough money to keep the family going on. I have no help although the two oldest children are now helping. My husband helps as much as he can on weekends. In the evening after all the children have been taken care of, my husband and I collapse in bed. On weekends there is even more work with the children because we have to occupy them at home. Sex is a problem because we have no time or energy for it. I am always scared of getting pregnant, in spite of all the birth control methods I have been using. I do not trust any of them except the pill, but it makes me gain weight, so I stopped them. I almost resent sex.

> *Q. Would you be freer to have sex in your old age after all the children are gone and after menopause so that you do not get pregnant? When your husband is retired, both of you will have plenty of rest, and you will have all the time for it.*
>
> *A. On the contrary, I plan to give it up altogether. I guess I wanted to have a large family like my mother, and that was the reason for having sex. Besides that I am not really interested in it. I find sex rather boring and even annoying.*
>
> *Q. What do you think your husband's attitude will be in this matter?*

A. I guess I will have to give in once in a while if he insists. But so far he has never made an issue of it.

* * *

One day I was discussing a tax return problem with my accountant. When we finished this professional discussion, we started discussing our personal interests in life and our hobbies. I mentioned that for many years I had been involved in a research project about sexuality in senior citizens. Although he was only in his mid thirties he expressed an immediate interest in the project. When I asked him the reason for his interest, his answer was he was curious to know what his sex life would be when he reaches sixty. We decided to conduct a full interview, the essentials of which follow:

Q. Can you summarize your current sexual life?

A. Sexual intercourse 2-3 times a week, my wife reaching orgasm about once a week.

Q. When you and your wife reach sixty, what do you think your sexual life will be?

A. I hope I will remain potent in order to satisfy my sexual desires and those of my wife. I may be concerned that my sexual desire may diminish while my wife's may not, or the reverse.

Q. Do you expect your sexual life to be different as a senior and if so, in what way?

A. It will be different for numerous reasons. Our sexual life will not be regulated by fear of pregnancy and contraception measures (no more withdrawal, no more condoms). My wife and I will not have to abstain during her menstrual periods because she will be post menopausal. Most of all, our three children will have moved out of the house and we will no longer be concerned about them hearing anything.

Q. Would the quality of your sexual act be different in any way? For instance, would your wife's body be less sexually attractive because of aging.
A. On the contrary, I expect the intensity of our relationship in general and our sexual relationship in particular to improve with time. We may have less sex, but not being busy with raising children or not being involved with professional activities, we will have more time for ourselves to know each other better, and to become more intimate. Our relationship will include sex but will go far beyond it.
Q. Are your parents still alive, and if so, what are their ages?
A. My father died 4 years ago at the age of 66 of a cerebral hemorrhage. My mother is now 68 years old and in good health.
Q. During the couple of years prior to your father's death, do you think or do you know if your parents were sexually active?
A. I suppose so, but I don't like to think about it and I am embarrassed to talk about it. In some way, I may think that sex for them may be inappropriate.
Q. How would you feel if your widowed mother tells you that she is going on a vacation trip with a man that she has been going out with lately?
A. My first reaction would be shock. On the other hand, she is lonely and more involved with my family than my wife and I would like. So, it could be a relief, in a way. I guess I would reason that it is her private life, and she is free to do what is best for her.

When discussing with the group of adults the issues related to senior sexuality, we did not include any relative or friend younger than 25 years of age, unless they were already married. We did not include these younger people because we felt that people under that age would be embarrassed by our personal questions. We also took note of the interviews that we considered non-satisfactory, such as those who were too embarrassed to discuss these problems in detail, and those who really did not know how to answer. We approached 1502 adults in all (569 males, 933 females) between the age of 25 and 55, all relatives of our senior population, in order to get their views on senior sexuality. Some young married couples with a widowed mother or father, would have wished the parent to remarry or at least have a companion, because they were fearful the parent may want to live with them. Some come to resent the intrusion of the parent in their life especially by the mother of a single daughter. This feeling often interfered with the children's interview and when we got the impression that this interfered with their objective opinion, the case was excluded from the study. We eliminated 449 adults or 30% who refused the interview or were considered unsatisfactorily interviewed and we tabulated only 1053 adults, whose interviews were considered satisfactory and deserved analysis.

In order to gain their confidence we discussed with them first their general impression on sexuality in senior age, and specifically how they envision their own sexuality when they reach senior age (Table 11). Among these 1053 subjects, 336 or 31.9% will abstain sexually in senior age for different reasons (religious, social, familial, personal). Others were fearful of being unable to perform (28.6%) or of not being able to satisfy the partner (21.7%). A surprising 17.2% will indulge more, sexually speaking, because they will be free of any obligations such as menses, pregnancy, privacy, or job. Sixteen percent did not know. In Table 11, almost all adults gave only one answer for each question: there were 1.12 answers for each question. This implies they have their mind set about their sexuality when seniors.

It appears therefore that about one-third of the adults plan to give up sex in senior age, about half would like to be sexually active but are afraid they will not be able to perform, and about one in six plan to indulge more in sex, and one in six did not know.

Table 11 also shows that adult men and women have different plans in their future sexual matter in general. Almost twice as many women (38.5%) than men (21.3%) plan to give up sex. Men are twice as fearful than women of not being able to perform. About the same number of men and women, one in six, plan to indulge more, sexually speaking.

We have not been able to delve into the reasons why so many adult women plan to give up sex when they reach senior age, because the more personal our questions became, the more we met resistance. But the immediate impression was that the non-orgasmic and generally non-satisfied women, plan to give up sex. Many of them consider it an obligation, especially the older adult woman and their plan is to free themselves from this sexual “duty” when the appropriate time comes.

What Adults Think Senior Sexuality Should Be

Adult children are almost always ambiguous about their senior parents' sexuality. This is illustrated in the following two case histories.

I am a 35 year old woman, divorced with two children. My sexual life was not great when I was married and did not get better afterward. The couple of sexual affairs I had since ended up miserably. Now I am busy with my job and raising my children. I date rarely and I even tried a lesbian relationship. I had no interest in it. When I am short of male companions and become restless, I occasionally masturbate in bed or when taking a shower. Somehow I always thought that my parents who now are 70 years old had peacefully retired and I never though of them having any kind of sexual activity. Was I in for a surprise! There was one day a serious incident when two years ago I went to spend a few days with my parents in Florida where they retired. One morning during my visit, I got up early to go shopping and told them I would be back in the afternoon. Fifteen minutes later I realized I forgot my credit card and drove back to get it. This is how I reconstructed the events afterwards. They took advantage of my absence to have sex. At the moment of his orgasm my father was rather noisy and I guess my mother was noisy too when about to reach her own climax at the same time. I heard both of them screaming and rushed upstairs to their bedroom, thinking that they were fighting and my father was physically abusive. Under no circumstances could I have realized that they were sexually active, both of them orgasmic and at the same time. I confess that I do not recall having had such an experience. Anyway I do not know what came over me, but I started to scream at them. I called them sexual perverts and insisted they go for therapy so that they learn how to act their age. I calmed down later on, but never recovered completely. A few days later my mother told me that she and my father are always sexually active the way I saw them. I still cannot comprehend that my parents who are twice my age, have a better sexual life than I do. I am still convinced that there is something wrong with them.

* * *

This 35-year old female physician was never married, had no children, and had one abortion. She refused to give details of her sexual life except that she is going out with somebody and uses birth control pills. For the time being at least, they are not planning any marriage. She insists that she likes her independence and is not interested in having children. However, she occasionally takes her brother's children to the amusement park on Sundays; she gets impatient with them after a couple of hours and is relieved to return them to their parents afterwards.

She is tall, nice looking, and uses very elaborate make up. When I asked her how she envisions her sexual life after the age of 55 she expressed tremendous anxiety. What would happen to her skin, would wrinkles appear all over her face, how long would her naked body be sexually attractive to her boyfriend. I made things worse when I asked her how she conceives her sexual life at the age of 70. She will fight to stay youthful for as long as possible, using physical exercise, massage, spas, and of course, plastic surgery. When I talked about 80, she definitely insisted that she did not want to live that long, although as a physician she knew she could easily reach that age. She does not expect sex at that age. Her mother is 60 years old, divorced, and at ease financially. She always wears excessive makeup, to the point of sometimes embarrassing her son and daughter. She spends a fortune on her hair, hands and toe nails, is always spending time on massages and health spas. She just had her third plastic surgery for a breast reduction. She previously had liposuction. She and her brother have talked about it and her brother has talked to his mother and asked her to act her age. She never did. Her mother has dated many people, some much younger than her. Her mother calls it 'women's liberation.' She presently lives with a man four years younger. Yes, her mother is sexually active and is open about it. But she never asked the details. She terminated the conversation as she was becoming more and more embarrassed.

Table 12 studies specifically the position of the young and adult toward the sexuality of their current senior relatives. The same 1502 were approached in this matter. Again, about 30% refused to cooperate or were unsatisfactorily interviewed. About 70% (1061) cooperated fully, of which 383 were men and 678 were women.

It should be noted that in Table 11, we received barely more than one answer (1.12) for each question. In Table 12, we got a little less than two answers (1.97) for each question. This implies that adults are more unsettled about what sexuality should be for their senior relatives, than what it should be when they become seniors themselves.

A little more than half (52.9%) think that their senior relatives should abstain completely. About one-fourth (24.9%) think they should refrain from it, another fourth (25.5%) think the seniors should have the same sexual activity as adults, and 9.3% think they should have more sex because they are free from any inhibition. Finally, 29.4% think it is up to the seniors to decide what they should do, and 19.2% did not have any answer. It is to be noted that 35.6% were embarrassed in discussing sexuality of their senior relatives.

Table 12 also shows that adult men and women have different concepts concerning sexuality of their senior relatives:

60% of adult women and only 40% of adult men think the seniors should abstain. Twice as many women (30.2%) than men (15.4%) think that at least they should be discreet about it. Slightly more men (30.3%) than women (22.7%) think it is the same as adults, and 12% of men and 7.7% of women think it could be more. Also 37.6% of men and 24.8% of women think that it is up to them. Finally, 40% of adult women are more embarrassed to discuss the subject than 28% of men.

In comparing Tables 11 and 12, it appears that current adults are more severe, sexwise, about their current senior relatives than they are about themselves when they reach senior age: only 31.9% of current adults plan to give up sex in senior age, but 52.9% think that their senior relatives should abstain. Similarly, 17.2% of current adults think they will indulge more sexually when they reach senior age because of more freedom, but they are willing to give the same freedom to only 9.3% of their current senior relatives. It is the old saying: "do as I say, not as I do." At any rate, it is obvious that there is some similarity between what adults wish they do when seniors and what they think seniors should do.

It should be recognized however that the current adult generation, mostly the younger ones, are willing to let the seniors decide for themselves what to do sexwise: 29.4% leave it up to them, more men (37.6%) than women (24.8%).

Children's Knowledge of Their Parents' Sexual Activity

I am now a 68 year old male. I retired four years ago. I worked all my life in a book store, children's section. I was frequently exposed to mothers' children and the opportunity for sexual affairs were frequent. My wife died of ovarian cancer fifteen years ago and since then I had numerous affairs and sometimes I had more than one affair at the same time. My two children, who are now grown up, always have known me as a womanizer. Honestly speaking, I always like to brag about it and until now I like to keep that reputation. It always boosts my ego when my son and/or daughter ask me: "What has been your last adventure lately?"

Something happened to me two years ago. When I had sex with a woman I started to have heart palpitations with a feeling of dread and anxiety. It got worse and worse and I had to stop sex. I saw all kinds of doctors and took all kinds of medications with limited results. Finally, my cardiologist suggested that I stop having sex altogether, which I did and I now feel much better. However, I did not want to destroy my reputation as a "senior playboy." I kept behaving the same way in front of everybody, and also bragged about my latest imaginary adventure, especially in front of my son who "looks up" to me in this matter. He still admires me for it and is almost jealous.

About 90% of the approached adults were the children of our senior population. The other 10% were siblings, distant relatives or just friends. In Table 13 we asked the adult children what accurate information they have regarding the sexual activity of their senior parents. When we approached these adult children we never identified their parents in order to guarantee anonymity and elicit confidential information. There were 965 adult children that were approached in this matter. About 10%

refused to cooperate or were unsatisfactorily interviewed. This left us with 870 adult children that were currently interviewed; 302 men and 568 women. The questions asked were very simple, and could be answered yes or no:

1. Is your parent (father or mother) sexually active?
2. Do you suspect that he/she is sexually active?
3. Do you doubt he/she is sexually active?
4. Is your parent, to the best of your knowledge, sexually inactive?
5. You do not know.

Of course we wished we could have verified the veracity of these answers by comparing with the senior parent's answer, but we never did it to respect confidentiality and anonymity. As will be seen later, the answer could be assumed indirectly.

We felt that only adult children could be asked such information about their parents because otherwise it could be considered invasion of privacy. Only one answer per adult son/daughter was considered. There were approximately two daughters for each son that answered.

About one-third had no knowledge whatsoever of what their parents were doing sexually speaking. About another third were adamant that their parents were not sexually active. The last third was more or less equally divided between those who were sure they had sex, those who suspect it, and those who doubt it.

The above averages, however, combine the responses of the sons and daughters that were put together. Table 13 also shows that the responses of the two genders are markedly different. The daughters believe more in the sexual abstention of their parents than do the sons. Among the sons, 19.2% believe and 13.6% suspect sexual activity of their senior parents, while, among daughters the figures are only 7.2% and 9.2%

respectively. Among the sons only 19.5% believe in their sexual abstention, while 38.4% of the daughters believe so. The general impression we got was that the adult sons were more objective and rational in their evaluation, while the daughters were more subjective and emotional in their response. We had at least eleven daughters who expressed anger at the idea that their (not married) parent could be sexually active.

In Table 14, we asked our sexually active senior population if their children were aware of their sexual activity. While Table 13 helps us understand the reaction of the adult children to their senior parents' sexuality, Table 14 helps us understand the senior parents' reaction to the children's knowledge that they are sexually active. Table 13 is an adult children's response and Table 14 is a senior parent's response.

There were 1402 seniors, 931 men and 471 women, that were heterosexually active (these data come from Table 17 that will be discussed later on). The questions asked were very simple and could be responded with a yes or no answer. Only one answer per senior was expected:

1. Your adult child(ren) know you are sexually active
2. Your adult child(ren) suspect you are sexually active
3. Your adult child(ren) doubt you are sexually active
4. Your adult child(ren) do not know you are sexually active
5. You do not know if your children are aware that you are sexually active

On some occasions, the senior parents have passed on to their children, directly or indirectly, the information about their sexual activity. On other occasions, it was the children who asked the information from their parents, and the parents responded their own way. Finally, there were cases where the parents did not know how the children got the information. In 21.7% the senior parent knew and in 17.7% they suspected that their children were aware of their senior parents sexuality. In 6.4% they doubted the children knew anything and in 38.8% they were sure the children did not know anything. Finally, in 15.4% of the time the senior parents had no idea about their children's knowledge of their parent's sexual activity. These figures combine the responses of senior men and senior women.

When we separate the responses of the senior men from the senior women, the figures show that the senior parents have different opinions. First, senior women are much less willing to recognize that their sexuality is known (10.4%) or suspected (14.9%) by their children, while more senior men are willing to recognize it (27.4% and 19.1% respectively). Second, almost half of the senior women (48.2%) categorically state that their children are convinced that their parents are sexually inactive, while only about one-third (34%) of the senior men are of the same opinion. Finally, one senior woman in five (20.6%) and one man in eight (12.8%) have no idea if their children are aware of their active sexuality.

In summary, about 40% of sexually active seniors are willing to recognize that their children are aware of their sexual activity (one senior man in two and one senior woman in four). Almost 45% of these seniors deny that their children have such knowledge (more than half of the senior women and about one-third of the senior men). The rest, about 15%, do not know if their children have any knowledge of their sexual activity (one senior woman in five and one senior man in eight).

In Table 15, the senior citizens that are sexually inactive were asked if their children were aware of their sexual inactivity. The bulk of the seniors declared that their children were aware of their sexual inactivity. There are, however, two interesting details in this table: 27 or 10.5% of the senior men declared that their children were convinced that they were sexually active, while really they were not; and 39 or 4.7% of the senior women declared that their children were convinced that they were sexually active, while really they were not.

We could not go further in this problem of awareness of senior sexual activity in the children/parent relationship because we wanted to fully respect their anonymity. For instance, we did not know (and we did not ask) if the children referred to in this investigation (Tables 14, 15) were all part of our studied population. Also, in this reciprocal study of children/parent knowledge of senior sexuality we did not determine the sex of the parent out of respect for privacy and because we did not know if the parent was part of this investigation. Finally, we did not ask the children about the age of their parent for the same reason of anonymity. At no time did we ever tell a senior parent that their child or children were part of the investigation, nor did we ever tell a child that his/her parent were part of the investigation, although they frequently told each other.

For the above reasons, the cohorts of population referred to in Tables 11-15 do not always refer to the same population of adult children and senior parents, and cannot accurately be used for comparison. In order to be 100% accurate, one can draw conclusion from each table individually and not compare one to the other. However, the number of subjects in these tables is rather high: up to 1502 adult children, and up to 1495 senior parents. Therefore one can cautiously attempt to oppose and compare conclusions from one table to another and draw some conclusions, being aware of the above restrictions.

Senior Concern Regarding Outside Opinion About Their Sexuality

The general impression one gets is that sexuality in senior citizens on one side and sexuality in adult children on the other side do not exist independently and somehow influence each other. This is obvious in Tables 11 and 12, and even 14 and 15. It is also obvious that adult children try to determine and at least influence the sexuality of their senior parents. Also obvious, some seniors feel that they are judged and they should account for their sexuality to their children. This is obvious in Tables 14 and 15. Finally, senior men and senior women react differently toward their adult children in terms of their sexuality and reciprocally. This is obvious in all tables and one can conclude that some senior parents are open about their sexuality, some are indifferent if it is known, and some are hysterical that it could be known by their children. "Hiding" it from their children is more frequent with senior women than senior men, as seen in Tables 14 and 15. When carefully pondering on these five tables, one is reminded of the Oedipus complex that was extensively studied by Sigmund Freud in the beginning of the last century and that has been so popular and fashionable during the last century among psychoanalysts. Briefly, Freud described some unconscious attraction of sexual nature between mother and son, between father and daughter, and this was associated with hidden aggression. This Freudian concept is not as popular anymore, but remnants of it can be found in Tables 11-15. It is unfortunate that Freud concentrated his study on the young and adult: he could have found as much if not more material in seniors. Deep psychoanalysis in older people has never interested psychoanalysts and there is barely any research on it. Senior sexuality could be a field for very interesting psychoanalytic research.

In Table 16, we approached the problem more directly. We asked all the seniors investigated in this study if they consider that there is an outside interference in regard to their sexuality. In a way this Table 16 is complementary to Table 12. Table 12 tells us what the outside world thinks the seniors should do in regard to their sexuality, while Table 16 tells us the response and the concern of the seniors to the outside world. In Table 12 the adults give an opinion. In Table 16, the seniors give an opinion. A total of 2722 seniors were interviewed in this matter, 1239 senior men and 1483 senior women (data taken from Table 17, as will be seen later). It should be specified, however, that the two cohorts are not the same: for instance in Table 12 the cohort of the 1502 adults that were approached gave their opinion on the sexuality of seniors in general and not necessarily on the cohort of the 2722 seniors investigated here; reversely in Table 16, the cohort of the 2722 seniors gave their opinion of the general adult population and not necessarily on the cohort of the 1502 adults that were approached. Again, the reason we proceeded in this manner is to respect full privacy of the interviewees without allowing seniors and adults to identify each other as parents and children. To compare Tables 12 and 16 may not be mathematically accurate but the number of interviewees is so high that the two tables can be juxtaposed and compared with statistical accuracy.

Table 16 shows that the senior population believes that the adult population think they should abstain completely from sex in a little less than one-third (30.3%) of the cases, they should restrain and be discrete about it in one case in seven (15%), they should have the same sexuality as adults in one-third of the cases (33.7%), they should increase in very few instances (3.6%), and that it is up to them in one-third of the cases. Finally, one senior in six (17.6%) does not know what the adult population thinks.

To be noted many senior answers were ambiguous and some gave more than one answer: 1.43 answers per senior.

On further analysis, Table 16 shows that senior men and women give markedly different answers concerning the adult opinions. For instance, twice as many senior women than senior men believe that the general adult population want them to abstain. Twice as many senior men than senior women believe that the general adult population wants them to have the same sexual activity as any other age. Finally, twice as many senior men than senior woman believe that the general adult population recognizes their right to make their own decisions. It appears that senior men believe in more sexual activity and more freedom in deciding about it.

It appears that the general adult population is stricter about senior abstention than the seniors would like. Table 12 shows that 52.9% of the adult population would recommend sexual abstention for seniors, while seniors themselves see only 30.3% as a recommendation. The same discrepancy between the two tables is found in other items: sexual restraint, freedom in sexual decision, etc. The final impression is that the general population is not too aware of the sexual liberation of the senior population and that the senior population is trying to send the message of liberation to come.

General View of Senior Sexuality

One day, as a resident training in obstetrics and gynecology, I had a 60-year old female patient who was referred to the gynecological clinic because she complained of vaginal bleeding and pain in the vaginal area. In women of this age, this complaint is ominous of possible gynecological cancer. I looked at her history and learned that she was a school teacher, single, and never had sexual relations. It was obvious that she was a typical spinster, dignified, borderline hostile and rather reluctant to provide any detail or to be thoroughly examined. At any rate I performed a complete physical examination including speculum examination, Pap smear, a vaginal examination, and biopsy in the bleeding area. The last part of the examination was rather embarrassing to the patient to say the least because she was obviously a virgin and had never had a vaginal examination previously. After she put her clothes on, she sat in front of me, angry, perplexed and wondered what was the purpose of all these examinations and what she considered an invasion of her private body. I calmly answered that we had to wait for the report of all the tests. At the next visit, the result of the biopsy showed that she had a cancer of the vulva (entrance to the vagina). She needed an extensive and mutilating surgical procedure, with a recovery period in the hospital that extended for one month. She turned out to be a warm person after all. We became very friendly during that period and called each other by our first names. I took care of her dressings each and every day. After discharge she needed periodic check ups every three to six months for the rest of her life. When I finished my residency program, she followed me in my private office for her check ups. One day during one of her check ups, she embarrassingly told me that she had masturbated all her life and wanted to know if that was responsible for her cancer. I reassured her that there was no relation whatsoever, that it was practiced by many women who did not have a sexual partner, and even by those that did have one, and that I had recommended this procedure to many women during my career.

One day she made a special visit to my office to announce that at the age of 65 she was getting married! Her future husband was about the same age, a widower, a colleague teacher in the same school, and he had made it clear to her that he wanted to be sexually active. While she did not mind, she wanted to make sure that it was feasible in view of her extensive surgery. All she needed was a minimal surgical procedure to remove the scar around the vaginal orifice and to enlarge the vaginal entrance, procedures I performed. She apprehensively 'submitted' herself to the sexual penetration, which became easier and easier. Six months later, she reported to me what appeared to be, from her description, a sexual climax. She described her husband as loving, kind, patient, skilled. Seven years later, her husband died of a heart attack, ending what she considered a very happy and sexually active married life.

A year later she entered a retirement home made up of senior citizens who were mostly in their seventies and where her sister had already been living for a couple of years. At that time I shared with her the purpose of a study which I wanted to get involved in, the study of sexuality in senior citizens. Would she participate in this study? She immediately rebuffed me, citing all kinds of religious, moral, social, and personal objections. I asked if she believed that our sexual discussions had brought her any help in her life. "Oh, definitely" was her answer. "Do you think that other senior people would be helped with such discussions?" "Oh, yes" was her answer, "and I already know a few people in the retirement home where I live who know my history and would benefit from such discussions." We had a few more meetings on that matter and she then decided to cooperate fully. This was the first subject of my 3396 series of cases about sexual activity in senior citizens. She was highly intelligent, well organized, and very social. She and her sister belong to all the committees in their community and managed to arrange many interviews which I personally conducted. We even conducted 'negative' interviews, and by that I mean I interviewed people who refused to discuss sexual matters and the reason for their objections. We also tabulated the people in the retirement home who were handicapped physically (bed ridden, wheel chair) or mentally (dementia, Alzheimer disease) handicapped. The result was that we were able to tabulate the sexual profile of practically the entire community, with special tabulation for those who declined the sexual interview. This was my first complete series on the subject of sexuality in senior citizens. I perfected the technique of approach in this community and I subsequently applied a similar technique in other communities, making sure that the profile of these communities varied in order to get a wide view of the different aspects of sexuality in the senior population at large.

After having eliminated the seniors who refused to or could not be interviewed, we had complete interviews with 2722 seniors, 1239 men and 1483. Tables 17, 18, 19 present the sexual profile of these senior citizens. From the sexual point of view, we recognized four categories of sexualities:

Heterosexuality
Homosexuality
Masturbation
No sexual activity

Heterosexuality occurs when individuals of opposite sex are involved in coitus, i.e., penetration of erect penis into the vaginal cavity, numerous thrusts and ejaculation for the man and climax (a different word for female orgasm) for the woman. We distinguished two types of heterosexuality. First, the orgasmic sexuality as just described and characterized by full orgasm in the senior man and full climax in the senior woman. The seniors do not have to reach orgasm-climax at each coitus and, when they reach it, it does have to be at the same time. As long as the senior man states that he has full erection, complete vaginal penetration, numerous thrusts, and full ejaculation, we considered him orgasmic. As long as the senior woman reaches her own climax with spasm over her whole body, numerous vaginal spasms and complete release afterwards, we considered her also orgasmic. We will see later that climax in women is much more difficult to define and to reach than male orgasm. At any rate, mostly in the senior population, orgasm and climax are not always easily reached. Many times coitus is poorly orgasmic and even non-orgasmic in the male: poor erection, difficult and limited penetration, limited thrusts with the coitus interrupted without ejaculation, and limited or no ejaculate. On the female side, limited or absence of climax is frequent, as the woman can be purely passive and not even attempting to reach climax. In Table 17, we call this kind of limited coitus, in the senior man and in the senior woman, poorly orgasmic or non-orgasmic, and we will use these last two words (poorly orgasmic and non-orgasmic) interchangeably.

Among the total of 2722 senior subjects that were interviewed, 1402 or 51.5% were heterosexually active, of which about two-thirds (911 subjects) were orgasmic and the other third (491 subjects) were poorly or non-orgasmic. There were however tremendous differences between senior men and senior women in terms of sexual activity and orgasmicity.

Among the 1239 senior men, 931 or 75.1% were heterosexually active: about three quarters among them (721 subjects) described what could be called orgasmic sexuality; the other quarter (210 subjects) were poorly and/or non-orgasmic and considered their sexual life non-satisfactory, in spite of repeated attempts. Among the 1483 senior women, only 471 or 31.8% declared themselves heterosexually active and even among these 471 heterosexually active senior women, only 190 (12.8%) among them were really reaching climax, while the other 281 (19%) were poorly orgasmic or had a purely passive attitude during coitus.

We had only three homosexual males and no homosexual females in our series. This number is rather low, although it is known that homosexuality is much less frequent among seniors than among the younger generation. It is also possible that many seniors who live in a closed community would prefer it not to be known, since seniors belong to the "old school" which frowns upon homosexuality. It is likely, and even certainly possible that the number was higher, but they refused interviews or classified themselves in a different category than homosexual. At any rate the number of senior homosexuals is so low that this will be excluded from the statistical study.

There were 224 cases (8.2%) of masturbation. But the difference between senior men and senior women was noticeable. There are three times as many masturbatory senior women (11.9%) than senior men (3.9%). Actually the percentage of masturbating senior men is the same as in adulthood, while the number of masturbating senior women more than doubled. The issue of masturbation will be discussed in a subsequent chapter.

Finally, 40.1% of seniors had no sexual activity. Here again there was a marked gender difference. Almost three times as many senior women (56.3%) than senior men (20.7%) abstain from sex.

All the above issues will be discussed separately in subsequent chapters.

Variations With Age of Senior Heterosexuality

I am 84 years old, widower for the last ten years. My wife and I were sexually active until she passed away suddenly of a heart attack. I abstained sexually for six months after she died, then I got involved with a widowed lady about ten years younger than I am. In the beginning of our relationship we were sexually active about three times a week. It has slowly decreased over the years and now it is only once every week or two. She does not reach climax anymore and is now rather passive during coitus. But she never objects to our sexual intimacy and even seems happy that I find her sexually attractive. My relationship with her has not changed however and we enjoy each other's company tremendously. She has her own children and I have my own and we all now form a big family. She is an excellent cook, and she knows how to save money without us being deprived of anything. I may be selfish when I say that I hope I will die first. I would not know what to do if I am a widower again. We wanted to get married, but people made so many jokes about it that we gave up the idea. We are also concerned that if one of us dies after we get married, it may create inheritance problems for our children.

Sexual activity in seniors varies with their age (Table 18 and Figure 3). The youngest seniors have a sexual activity similar to the oldest adult as will be seen later. On the average, 75.3% of senior males are heterosexually active, fully orgasmic or poorly orgasmic. Between 55 and 59 years of age, 89.1% of senior men are sexually active. Then there is a slow irregular decline and after 85 years of age it is only 38.9%. A similar decline is observed among senior women. On the average 31.8% of senior women are sexually active. Between 55 and 59 years of age, 33.5% of senior women are sexually active. Then there is a slow and irregular decline and after 85 years of age, it is only 21.2%. The decline of sexual activity in senior women is much more irregular than in senior men and in fact there is an upsurge (40.7%) in the 65-69 years of age group, and a sharp decline in the 70-74 years of age group. In order to explain the upsurge and decline, we considered the possibility that some women in that age group of 70-75 declared themselves younger than they really were. Of course these can be nothing else but expected variations in view of the relatively small number of senior women in some age group and one could be satisfied with the simple and statistical conclusion that out of 1483 senior women, a little less than one-third among them are sexually active, and their sexual activity is more or less evenly and irregularly spread among these different ages.

Many conclusions can be drawn from these figures, however. Among senior men, the sexual activity appears striking since (considering all ages) three quarters of them are sexually active and 38.9% of them are still active after 85. To be noted also is that, percentage wise, senior women (31.8%) are much less sexually active than senior men (75.3%). Although there is a slight and irregular decline with age, this low sexual activity in women has a tendency to persist in spite of advanced aging: on the average only 31.8% of senior women are sexually active, but the figure maintains itself at 21.2% after 85.

Table 18 combines all types of heterosexuality, orgasmic, poorly orgasmic, or non-orgasmic. Table 19 distinguishes orgasmic heterosexuality from other types of heterosexuality. They will be studied separately later on.

One could conclude that sexual activity after 85 years of age, 38.9% in men and 21.2% in women, is surprisingly elevated. One should not conclude that the percentage of seniors who are sexually active is high because this percentage is in relation to the 2722 investigated seniors and not in relation to the 3396 approached seniors, of which 20% are sexually inactive.

Kinsey et al. reported similar figures in senior men, but much higher figures in senior women. Their number of reported cases was rather small, and, besides, they dealt only with volunteers up to 60 years of age. Ours is the first large series reported in the literature on the subject, at such advanced ages.

Masturbation is infrequent among seniors: 48 out of 1236 senior men (or 3.9%) and 176 out of 1483 senior women (or 11.9%). It is irregularly steady at different ages. Masturbation is summarized in Table 19 and will be investigated in a separate chapter.

Finally, a sizeable number of seniors are sexually inactive (Table 19): 20.8% of senior males and 56.4% of senior females abstain. Surprisingly, the abstention figures do not show a progressive increase with age: there is a very irregular increase of abstention in senior men, and a high but steady level of abstention in senior women.

Variation in Frequency of Coitus Among Sexually Active Seniors

I always find it amazing how frequent sexuality can be even in very advanced age. It is also surprising how little this is known. This is shown in the following two cases.

I am 85 years old, a widower for 30 years and I retired from my job as an accountant at the age of 66. I want to be honest and declare that I have been a womanizer all my life and still am. Even when my wife was alive I had numerous affairs and very often more than one at a time. My wife never knew this other aspect of my life or, at least, pretended not to. After her death I kept the same life style. I am at ease financially and I like to go on cruises, or any kind of vacation trip. I do that a few times a year, and almost never with the same lady. I learned the hard way never to go out with a woman much younger than I am, for the simple reason that they expect too much out of you in terms of sex, money, and entertainment. On the opposite, senior ladies expect less out of you and to offer a lady a cruise or a vacation trip, all expenses paid, is more than they can ask for. In fact, very often the lady proposes to share the expenses but I always refuse because I always want to behave like a gentleman. Six months ago I met the lady I am currently with. She is ten years younger than I am and just as desirous for sex as I am. We got sexually involved two to three times a week and she reaches climax at least half of the time. For each affair I say to myself I am going to settle down with this one; and so, with this last one I again plan to settle down!

* * *

I am 81 years old , a widow for the last eleven years. My husband died from a broncho pneumonia that got complicated. Up to his death we were sexually active on the average of twice a week and we were both orgasmic most of the time. He kept at his job as a financial advisor to the end. On my side, I love playing piano. After my husband passed away, I quickly understood that, widow or no widow, sex is an important part of my life. I have to confess that neither my husband nor I had been faithful to each other during our married life. He had occasional relationships with office secretaries and, on that, I closed my eyes. On my side, I got involved for many years with my piano teacher and another time with a member of the orchestra I played in. Anyway, one year after my husband passed away I got involved with a man ten years younger than I was (I lied to him about my age), and we have been together since. My sexual life is now the same as it used to be with my husband before he passed away, i.e. about twice a week and full climax. My companion is very patient and very skilled in this matter and he will never approach me sexually unless I consent to it or ask for it. We have occasional periods of abstention, mostly when one of us is away or involved with children. He lives with me in my house and I pay almost all the expenses. I do not mind because I am more at ease financially than he is and, anyway, I wonder why the man should always support the woman in this kind of situation. In view of what I see around, compared to other women of similar age, I have a good life. I also consider myself very lucky because of the tremendous understanding and support I find from my two children. They are both very attached to me and are grateful to the man who makes me so happy.

* * *

Table 20 and figure 4 describe the frequency of coitus among the sexually active seniors. On the man's side, the average is 2.4 sexual acts a week. There is a steady decline with age from 3.2 sexual acts a week among the 55-59 group, down to once a month after 85 years of age. These, however, are average figures and the variations of performance among individual men were tremendous: some senior individuals were having coitus every day, others once every two to three months. The highest recordings were eight senior citizens between the ages of 60 and 69 who had daily coitus, and one eighty six year old man with bi-weekly sexual activity.

On the woman's side, there is a similar trend except that among sexually active senior women the average is only 1.6 coitus a week, while in sexually active senior men it is 2.4. Also in senior women the decline with age is much slower from 1.9 a week in the 55-59 range to 0.6 a week after 85 years of age. It appears that senior men start their sex life with a high frequency, but lose it progressively, while senior women start at a lower rate but lose it more slowly.

In order to go deep in this issue, we separated truly orgasmic from poorly orgasmic men, and orgasmic from poorly orgasmic and non-orgasmic women by similar age group. These data are presented in Table 20.

On the male side, orgasmic frequency is on average much higher: 2.9 coitus a week, with a range of sexual activity from daily to once every two weeks. With age, the frequency diminishes very slowly with an average of twice a week in the younger group (range from daily to twice a week) to every two weeks after 85 years of age (range from twice a week to once every two weeks).

On the male side, the figures for poor orgasm are much lower and they decline with age much faster, with a range of two weekly attempts to one every three months.

On the senior woman's side, the range of orgasmicity is much higher, from almost daily on the high side to almost weekly on the low side. The characteristic of orgasmic senior women is that the frequency of sexual orgasm stays high up to the eighties.

Senior women without orgasm, on the contrary, remain with a low frequency from twice a week to once every three months. In the young seniors it ranges from three times to once a week and, in the eighties, it goes from once a week to every quarter.

The reasons for these extreme variations will be studied subsequently.

Comparing Sexual Activity Before and After 55

The following two cases of a senior man and a senior woman show how a life of misunderstanding can reflect on senior sexuality, and on senior life in general.

I do not understand what happened to my sexual life. My wife and I are about the same age of 77. We have been married for 53 years. I started as a bank teller and the last ten years before retirement I became manager in a small bank. My wife always had a part-time job in a big department store. We had only one child, a son, who has his own family. We are both now retired but our relationship has changed dramatically sexually speaking. During all our working years our sexual life was routine. Coitus about twice a week, me mostly asking and her most of the time barely consenting. In the mid-fifties, after her change of life and after our son left home, she suddenly changed. She consented to sex only when she was in the mood for it, which was not very frequent. Besides, she insisted on what she called "preparation" and requested an elaborate presex procedure I never heard of and that most likely she picked up in a woman's magazine or from some other women in the beauty parlor. I try to follow her in these requests but thanks God, she does not ask for sex that often. It is not that I object so much but I feel very strange being involved in sexual procedures at the level of my great grandchildren (my son is grandfather to two teenagers). As I struggle to keep my orgasm going and as I become fearful of approaching impotence, my wife is discovering more and more sexual climax. Do you have any advice?

Answer: Have you tried Viagra?

* * *

I am 68 years old and my husband retired about two years ago. Our three children all left the house, the two daughters are married and the youngest the son, a young lawyer, is still single and lives by himself. My husband and I sill live in the same big house and there is no more activity in it. I suspect that we are both bored and we are getting on each other's nerves. My husband does not understand that our lives have changed since he retired, after the children were gone, after I got my menopause. He used to request sex whenever he liked it, never caring about me. He never understood that I was just complying to his request, whether I was desirous or not. Now we have sex only when I want it too, which means both of us have to want it. Now our sexual activity has dropped between once a week to once every two weeks, which is my range of desire. I still comply to his requests but not as frequently as before, although he has threatened to look for sex outside. The situation has become delicate because I resent sex more and more.

Q: Have you tried marriage counseling?

A: No. I do not feel it is necessary.

The 2722 seniors (1239 men and 1483 women) whose sexuality has been studied in the previous tables have also been asked to give information about their previous sexuality during adult life before they reached 55 years of age. Their adult sexuality is presented in Table 21 and is compared to their current senior sexuality.

On the male side, the number of sexually active subjects decreased by about 10%, from 1041 sexually active adults to 931 sexually active seniors. But the number of subjects with good orgasmicity decreased by 22% from 924 to 721, while the number with poor or no orgasmicity increased from 117 to 210 (an 80% increase). Homosexuals went down from 9 to 3, and masturbation cases from 57 to 48. Individuals with no sexual interest (mostly impotent) increased by 58% from 114 to 180 and those with no sexual partner increased from 18 to 77 (an increase of 328%). In summary, comparing adult men to senior men, there is a slight to moderate decrease in different sexual activities, and a slight to moderate increase in poor or no sexuality.

On the female side, the changes are more or less in the same direction but much more drastic. The number of sexually active senior women drops by more than half (55%) compared to only 10% in men. Orgasmicity drops about equally, 20.2% in women and 22% in men. But it is in non-orgasmicity or poor orgasmicity that senior women and senior men are different. While the number of non-orgasmic or poor orgasmic men increases from 117 to 210, some senior men continue to struggle and to hold on to a declining potency. Senior women, on the contrary, give up non-orgasmicity in about two-thirds of the cases, from 816 to 281. It appears that many of them prefer to give up sex rather than going on with non-orgasmicity which does not interest them anymore. We will return tot his point later on. Some who still are interested in orgasm but have no partner turn to masturbation which more than doubles from 70 to 176 cases. As a consequence also, the senior women who give up sex for no interest more than doubles. Finally, the number of senior women with no partner increases from 216 in adulthood to 506 in seniorhood. To be noted, these 506 senior ladies said they have no partner but do not necessarily say they miss a sexual partner. We will return to this point later on. In summary, comparing adult women to senior women, there is a marked drop in sexuality, but a much less noticeable drop in orgasmicity and much more noticeable in non-orgasmicity. In addition, more senior women turn to masturbation, or give up sex altogether. Finally, the number of senior women with no partner more than doubles.

This difference between orgasmic and non-orgasmic seniors may appear high. This is so because our definition of orgasm was very strict: full erection and ejaculation following several thrusts in males and all the criteria for female climax with tonic contractions, resolution and successive vaginal spasms. The orgasm had to occur at least every two weeks. To be noted is that many senior women declared themselves climactic while on further investigation it became obvious that they confused real climax with satisfaction of a different nature. This point will be elaborated upon later.

Masturbation Practice

I am now 71 years old. I have been a high-level executive in a woman's magazine all my life until I retired at the mandatory age of 65, but I still am a consultant working part-time. My sexual life has been hectic during my whole career. I got married at the age of 25 and divorced my husband four years later, no children. I do not know how to say it, but it was assumed as a part of my job to get sexually involved with different men I was exposed to professionally. It was almost a standard story: first a purely business relationship, then "may I invite you for dinner," then when I was driven home the usual "would you like to come up for a while ?" Whether the man was married or not, we ended up in my bed half of the time, and the relationship could end right there after the first night or be carried on for a while. As I aged and in spite of repeated plastic surgeries, these propositions became less frequent, although here and there there were occasional "hot sparks" with young or not so young executives. I did not mind this diminished frequency because I was becoming bored or even irritated with it. Either the man was interested only in a quick sexual affair and he could not wait to walk away immediately afterward, or I could not wait to have him leave; or it was an interesting relationship and its mandatory termination, sooner or later, was becoming emotionally unbearable. The last interesting sexual affair I had five years ago left me so distressed that I decided it would be the last...

Anyway, parallel to this sporadic heterosexual life, at the age of 40 I developed a lesbian relationship with a colleague of mine. It lasted only one year and I had to stop it because of the gossip that was spreading in the office. At any rate, she initiated me in the art of masturbation, and until now I still continue with it. I always practice it almost every night unless there is a man around. Even then, when the coitus was not climactic, I completed it to full climax with my own fingers. Now and since the age of 66 my sexual activity is purely masturbatory. I practice it between daily to every third day, whenever I feel like it.. There is no pressure, no apprehension in satisfying anybody and it is always associated with some climax. Although I aged, I consider myself still sexually attractive since I still get propositions from mature gentlemen here and there. I always turn them down now.

Q: How would you compare the heterosexual climax you reached previously when you were younger, to the masturbatory climax you reach now on your own.

A: The heterosexual climax was much more intense and usually left me in a state of ecstasy for a whole day, while the climax with masturbation is less intense and short lived.

Q: Then why don't you search for a permanent relationship with a man about your age, since you said you still get propositions?

A. I will get too involved and I am afraid I am not up to it. To be permanently involved with a man is a total life involvement and not only a sexual involvement. Honestly, there would be too much involvement and I don't think I have the energy for it. I am satisfied the way things are. Why look for trouble.

Table 21 describes the practice of masturbation among our population of 2722 senior citizens (1239 males and 1483 females), and compares it to this practice in the same population before the age of 55. On the male side, it was minimal (4.6%) in adulthood and decreased slightly (3.9%) in seniorhood. On the female side, it was also moderate to minimal (4.7%) in adulthood, but it jumped to 11.9% in senior age; it more than doubled, it almost tripled.

The problem of masturbation is very difficult to discuss especially among senior citizens. Some of them associate it with sin, others with disgust or shame, and many consider it a failure, i.e., failure to secure the proper partner, and taking the easy way out to satisfy a biological urge.

There are a few explanations for the increase in masturbation among senior women. There is a marked shortage of available men for senior women and they therefore turn to masturbation. Quite a few senior men do not have the "biological" urge, become partially or totally impotent, prefer eating and/or drinking, enjoy the company of other men, but most of all they shy away from lonely senior women who are becoming more and more aggressive. As long as a men is running after a woman, the game may be interesting and stimulating. But with the reverse, it is the man who now runs away.

The other explanation is that the anatomy of the female body is predisposing to facilitate masturbation. I insist on this point, although many researchers disagree with me on this matter. Male masturbation is a very elaborate procedure that needs privacy, exposing one's genitals, the use of one and most of the time both hands, the frequent need of a lubricant, and it takes a relatively long time as it may not be always successful in terminating with ejaculation.

Masturbation in women is much simpler. Although many use their fingers with soap while taking a bath or a shower, others may not need their fingers at all. Rubbing the inner thighs one against the other is enough to lead to an orgasmic masturbation if the lady is in the proper mood. Privacy is not necessary. Some women have mentioned to me that they masturbate (without fingers) while bicycling or horseback riding. A lady mentioned to me that she did it frequently while using the old style sewing machine with a foot pedal. A lady supervising many women working in a large factory mentioned to me that she can pick up the women masturbating while at work. They do it just by rubbing her thighs rapidly against each other. No man can do that. I hope I have explained the reasons women masturbate more frequently than men.

There are some variants to masturbation. I call the one variant hetero-masturbation, in which as a preparation to coitus the male partner massages the clitoris of his female partner and/or the female partner massages the penis of her male partner. At least half of the sexually active senior population mentions such a procedure when they are specifically asked about it, although they indulge in it only occasionally.

Another variant, I call it additional masturbation, i.e., addition to regular coitus. The female partner massages her clitoris prior to coitus in order to facilitate her climax. Another variant of additional masturbation, not much talked about, is massage of the clitoris after coitus if and/or when the male partner withdraws without waiting for her to reach climax: the quick trips to the bathroom after male ejaculation without female climax sometimes have this purpose. These additional procedures have been mentioned by about 15 of the sexually active senior females.

There is also what I would call coital masturbation. Men and women are on their side, with the man facing the back of his female partner and performing vaginal entrance and coitus from the back (position #5, as one will see later). The male partner places his hand to the front of the female body and massages her clitoris at the same time as he is performing his thrusts. Some men do it with the hand between the female thighs in front of their penis. Some men manage to massage the clitoris of their partner even in the classical position of the man on top of the female partner and facing her: he has to be young senior, still vigorous and slim (position #1, see later).

Finally, some women manage to massage their own clitoris in the side to side position #5.

The reason I expanded on these variants of masturbation is

because they are much more frequent in seniors than in the adults or younger. I barely heard of them in the latter, while senior women mention them in 33 cases or 7%. I personally recommended with success these variants of masturbation to some senior women. My conclusion is that they deserve to be more known.

The anatomy and physiology of masturbation in females will be discussed in a later chapter.

Sexual Positions in Senior Age

While the mechanics of sexual activity are basically the same in adults and in seniors, some differences become evident as seniors advance in age. These differences stem from the principle that the senior citizen is physically weaker as he/she advances in age. Another reason is that seniors are more or less set in a preferred position. This is true for both sexes, but mostly the male.

The younger generation gets involved in elaborate preparations which can last an average of 15 minutes before the actual sexual act. This includes kissing, petting, touching breasts and genitalia. This necessary stimulation is used mostly by young men to induce a young woman to the sexual act and eventually to orgasm, for which the young woman might not be ready until properly prepared. Modern young women, however, can be very elaborate and knowledgeable in terms of preparation. One can also add that the younger generation is not fully skilled in terms of sexual techniques, and learn during preparation the best way to stimulate each other. Young men quickly learn that it is not easy to sexually arouse a woman and the quicker they learn the better.

For seniors it is completely different. Preparations are limited, if not nil. There is no such thing as a senior picking up at a party a woman who had no intention of a sexual encounter, and arousing her through kissing, petting, touching, and finally leading to the sexual act. Most, if not all the time, seniors are expert in sexual technique or there is nothing for them to learn from the sexual point of view, regardless if it is a spouse, companion, or prostitute. Sex in seniors is mostly planned, mostly on schedule, and there is nothing unexpected. Courtship, i.e., time between the first encounter and the sexual act is rather short. One main reason for such a short courtship is that the female partner more or less immediately makes her sexual intentions known and sometimes even makes the advance, thus cutting short all courtship and preparation for sex.

In this matter, female senior sexuality is rather simple, and completely different from the younger female generation who, from a sexual point of view, does not always know what they want and are tremendously inhibited because of fear of losing virginity, fear of painful sex, difficulties in dealing with bizarre sexual requests or sexual positions, fear of pregnancy, menstruation, venereal diseases, and so on. The senior woman has practically none of these concerns. Because it is 'pure' sex and because there is little unknown and little to be feared, she engages more freely in sex. If the senior woman is orgasmic she knows how to deal with the male and how to lead him to elicit her sexual orgasm. If she is not orgasmic, either she turns down the request or accepts the passive sexuality for motivations of her own. Senior women control and restrain themselves very well during sex. Be as it may, preparation that does not lead to sex does not interest them as much as before senior age.

The elaborate, prolonged, varied, and exhausting sexual performances, essentially seen in pornographic displays, are out of the question for seniors as their age advances further and further. Pornographic videos are commonly used by senior males, mostly in hotels but also at home, only for sex arousal but barely for learning any new sex technique. While most or all the positions seen in the young and adults are also seen in seniors, the order of frequency is completely different. In younger age, one sees the following positions by order of frequency (Table 22 and Figures 5, 6 and 7):

1. The customary position, viz. female on her back, man on top, facing each other

2. The reverse; female on top

3. Mounting, animal position, rear entrance to vagina, female

on hands and knees

4.Side to side, facing each other, legs crossing, or Japanese posture

5.Side to side, male facing back of female, rear entrance to vagina

6.Any combination of the above

The young and adults, especially the younger, prefer the customary position (#1), although the modern young and liberated female often request the reverse (#2). Mounting (#3) is sometimes indulged in the young. The side to side (#4) and the rear entrance to vagina (#5) are not the most popular in the young and adults and they are encountered only when the female partner is minimally involved. Sex while standing or sitting are exclusive positions of the young when taking a shower together, or getting sexually involved unexpectedly like at a party, in the park, or in a car. Most of all the young combine and prolong positions #1 and #2, alternating both or other positions. To be noted, however, is that the male adult sometimes objects to position #2 as he considers it an infringement on his 'macho' male dominance. Nudity is preferred by the young generation after they have known each other for a while.

I am 64 years old, divorced with two children. I divorced my wife 25 years ago. I am the co-owner of a summer camp and I still run it. It keeps me busy in the summer and I go to Florida in the winter, except for a couple of weeks in the winter during which I run the camp as a ski resort for children and some of their parents. I have been living with the same lady friend for the last twenty-five years. Until fifteen years ago our preferred sexual posture was, after the proper preparation, my lady friend lying on her back and me on top of her, facing her. We barely varied that position except when I was tired and still wanted sex, the role was reversed: she "prepared" me up to full erection and goes on top of me. Occasionally we mixed the two positions.

Starting fifteen years ago, I was easily getting tired when coitus lasted longer than usual and, besides, I started gaining weight which became more and more uncomfortable for my sexual partner. We started exploring other sexual positions and we found many suggestions in different women's and men's magazines. We now lie on our sides facing each other and crossing our legs. Since I usually lie on my right side, I put my left leg between her legs, with our bodies forming almost a right angle. Of course in this position there is less body contact but I manage a satisfactory penetration. We have sex about twice a week but my partner does not reach climax as often as she used to. She does not mind.

Both senior men and women are very concerned about the physical appearance of their bodies and concerned about physically looking old. This is the reason they keep on as much clothing as possible (pajamas) and expose only the part of their body necessary for sex.

In senior age, and even starting at the end of adulthood, the order of frequency is completely different (Table 22). To begin with, there is barely any variety during the sexual act as seniors mostly stick to only one position during the whole performance. Prolongation is also reduced to a couple of minutes, barely more, for the whole act, because the senior male tires quickly and/or the senior woman gets bored if not orgasmically involved. As seniors advance in age they look for sexual positions that relieve the female of male weight and that becomes more restful for the male.

Senior males start their senior age with position #1 (customary position) the most frequent. They use it less and less as they advance in age and in the seventies and eighties it is met only in one-third to one-fourth of the cases (Figure 5).

Senior females hang onto position #1 for much longer in advanced age where it is met in about half of the cases. It is a comfortable position for women but they have to give it up if the sexual partner is too heavy or takes too long to finish his sexual act. Some considerate male partners stay on their elbows and knees, thus sparing their female partner their full weight. They have to be slim and healthy.

Position #2, or female on top, is almost exclusively requested by orgasmic females up to the most advanced age, although isolated cases of poorly orgasmic males find it sexually stimulating in old age (Figure 5). To be noted, the senior female, in position #2, does not impose her weight on the male partner, because she is sitting most of the time, or on her arms forward on the bed.

Position #3, or mounting similar to animals, is seen only among the youngest seniors and disappears quickly with advanced age (Figure 5).

Position #4 (side to side, facing each other, Japanese posture), and more so position #5 (side to side, rear entrance to vagina) are definitely the preferred positions in senior age (Figure 6)

I am 70 years old and have been married to the same man for half a century. He has been and still is sexually demanding and we still have our daily intercourse in spite of our advanced age. To this day, I never turned down his requests because he always has been and still is good looking and a lot of women of all ages are still turning around him. I figured that the best way to keep him with me is to constantly occupy him with me, sexually speaking, so that he does not have to go anywhere else. Anyway, I would have settled for less sexual activity although I enjoy it sometimes and I reach climax here and there. For the last ten years I have become indifferent and even a little bored with sex, especially now that it takes him longer and longer to reach full erection and longer and longer to reach his orgasm; all that time I just want him to finish. A friend of mind with whom I discussed the problem suggested that we change position. He now approaches me from the back while we are both on our sides. What a comfortable position it is! Especially that my husband likes it too because he can stop whenever he wants without finishing the sexual act. For my part I can do what I want in that sexual position: I can rest, listen to music, read, watch TV. Sometimes I even forget that he is on my back and fall asleep. I would and I did recommend it to women who do not have much interest in sex but have to deal with a demanding sex partner.

In fact, for senior citizens positions #4 and #5 become the preferred and only position for an additional reason. Many senior sexual acts are of poor quality, i.e., passivity in the female and poor erection/no ejaculation in the male. As both partners get tired there is a tendency to get it over by giving up. In positions #1 and #2, one has to 'officially' recognize the impotence and give up the sexual act. But in positions #4 or 5, either one or both partners just has to slow down and stop the thrusts without changing position. One or both can even fall asleep. The point is that in these positions, the senior male can give up reaching ejaculation without changing position and, therefore, without losing face. Therefore, it is easier for the senior to attempt sex, even if poor erection and no ejaculation in these two positions.

Combination of positions, very frequent in young age, rapidly disappears in seniors (Figure 7).

We also discussed with seniors the duration of their coital act and the number of thrusts per coitus. The responses we got were haphazard, variable when the same question was asked more than once during the interview, and very often confusing. More often than not the interviewed senior did not know or was rather embarrassed to answer. The impression was that some seniors were capable of a prolonged coitus, others of a very short one and ejaculated immediately. Some thrusts were deep and frequent, others not so deep and not so frequent. No worthwhile tabulations could be made in this specific subject.

After Sex in Senior Citizens

During my years of counseling in my obstetrical and gynecological practice, I learned that an important aspect of sexual life is how the sexual partners feel toward each other after the sexual act has been terminated. After all, spouses and sexual companions do not spend their life having sex, which occupies only a small part of their life. The most important part of their common life is non-sexual, starting immediately after coitus, and the effect of their sexual life on their general life starts immediately after coitus. This is how humans are different from animals. Animals of opposite sex ignore each other as partners when not involved in coitus. Humans, differently, have to contend with each other even outside of their sexual activity.

We did this study comparatively by studying the post coital behavior of the adults and of our senior population (931 senior males and 471 senior females). Only heterosexually active adults and seniors were considered (Table 23). This table is limited to seniors who had a vivid recollection of their sexuality when they were adults.

How do I feel about my wife after we finish having sex? That is an interesting question and I never thought about it. Let us see, it depends. It has changed over the years. I remember when we were young, there was a lot of passion during sex. All we wanted to do was have sex, even a few times a day. We were exhausted afterward and I usually went to sleep. It was very important for me to arouse her sexually, and I was in no rush to ejaculate. We tried all kinds of positions, etc. Over the years it has changed. I do not have to prove anything to her: that I am very potent, virile. What I am she knows it by now. In bed, we watch a TV program together or we read a book, or we just talk, sometimes holding hands. Occasionally one of us expresses desire for sex and the other may agree or not: "I am too tired, I am sleepy, I do not feel like it, not tonight" and so on. The other does not make much out of it, does not feel angry or frustrated. After sex? Well, we stayed the way we were before or the same way we would be if we did not have sex. That is we keep watching the same TV program, or reading a book, or just talking, or holding hands, until one of us starts yawning, then we turn the light off and go to sleep. Sometimes, the following day we do not remember whether we had sex or not.

Q: Do you consider a time when you will stop all sexual activity?

A: Oh, yes. We even joke about it. I am now 73 years old and my wife is one year younger. I guess that within a few years sex will fade away and we will slowly forget about it. I am sure we will keep sleeping in the same bed, watching TV or reading a book, or just talking and holding hands until one of us falls asleep.

Q: Do you consider the time when one of you will pass away?

A: Yes, and last year I got scared after my wife had a mild heart attack. I wanted to give up sex, but she insisted on doing it. We just found a more restful and less stressing sexual position. If she passes away I will be lost. If I pass away first, I know she will readjust eventually.

Among men, there were striking differences between the young adult group and the senior group. The younger group are interested in prolonging coitus (83.8%) in changing positions during coitus and do their best to make sure that their female partner also reaches orgasm (53.5%). For some of them, however, orgasm and climax were the end, and they did not do much to extend the romance beyond orgasm: 33.1% wanted to be left alone, 26.8% even walked away, mostly when with casual encounters or prostitutes. Very few (12.5%) kept hugging the partner after ejaculation or had a feeling of loving ecstasy. Finally, one out of five (19.8%) were not clear in their answer.

The senior men definitely had a different post coital attitude. They also wanted to extend coitus but only half as often (39.3%) as young and adults. They just do not have the physical energy to extend it. They also want their partner to reach her climax but only in 22.8% of the cases and this for the same reason as above, i.e., lack of energy. Some seniors give up in the middle of coitus due to tiredness, diminished erection, or no ejaculation. However, contrary to the younger generation, they have a tendency to extend the post-coital romance more often: less often they want to be alone after orgasm (22.9%), they rarely walk out (12.6%) except with a prostitute, they are more relaxed and keep the relation casual (41.7%), and they are a little more often ecstatic about coitus (10.5%) than the younger. Almost all young-adults believe that their sexual life affects their general life, while only 22.9% of seniors do. Finally they are much less ambiguous when discussing the subject.

How do I feel after sex? I feel nothing. It is becoming routine, almost a bore and even an annoyance. I am now 70 years old and we still have sex because my husband still wants it and I want to please him because I love him. He has always been kind and considerate. If I do not feel like it, he does not insist. What I resent the most after having sex is that after he has finished he quietly relaxes and falls asleep, while I have to go to the bathroom to take a vaginal douche. This wakes me up completely and it takes me a good half hour listening to my husband snoring before I can go to sleep.

I may be selfish but I love it when we stay in bed for more than one hour, just talking, laughing, gossiping over the daily events, and finally falling asleep still holding hands and even embracing without any idea of sex.

Q: Do you still reach a climax?

A: Occasionally, and I always let him know ahead of time that I am in the mood. He becomes thrilled with it and for that night we recover our fountain of youth, just the way we were fifty years ago.

Among women, there were also noticeable differences between the young-adult on one side and the senior female generation on the other side in terms of their post coital feelings. The majority of the young and adults are definitely involved with their sexual life and it reflects on their general behavior starting immediately after coitus.

The majority of young-adult women (72.9%) also wanted to extend coitus up to climax, and also twice as frequently as senior ladies (40.6%). However, the frustration of the young group about not reaching orgasm was high (60%), while the senior ladies were much less frustrated (25.9%). Very few young adult women brush climax off their mind during coitus (12.1%), while 40.1% of senior ladies engage in coitus without planning any orgasm. Only 5.3% young-adult women are annoyed with sex and want to get it over, while four times as many senior ladies (21.9%) do. Only 7.8% of the younger group enjoy sex even without climax, while 10% of the senior women do. Finally, the majority of the young group (81.3%) think that their sexual life markedly affects their general life while only 36.1% of senior ladies do so. More young ladies are ambiguous about their answers (22.4%) than senior ladies (5.9%).

What can we conclude about these post coital behaviors when comparing adults and seniors and when comparing senior men and senior women? Let us clearly specify that Table 23 deals only with sexually active people, adults as well as seniors. First, sexual life is more important for the young and adult than for seniors. Therefore, lack of it affects the young and adult more than the senior. Let us not forget however that still almost one-fourth of sexually active senior men (22.9%) and more than one-third (36.1%) of sexually active women declare that their sexual life markedly affects their general life. It appears also that the young and adult women expect more from their sexual partners than do senior women. Finally, there is more "romance" and more post coital feeling among junior women than senior women. Seniors appear to be more casual about sex and are ready to slow it down and even do without it. We will see later that sex is not the most important thing that unites seniors, although it is so for some of them.

Sexual Profile in Married Senior People

My husband and I have been married for 47 years until he died last year of a brain tumor. Everything was alright until six months before he died when he started having trouble with his vision in the left eye. He refused surgery, developed all kinds of complications, then fell into a coma and died a week later. We had a fantastic life together. We had arguments, of course, and even had problems with one of our three children who has been in trouble with the law, but we overcame everything. When we retired 15 years ago (I am now 79) our attachment for each other remained the same until the day he died. As of the age of 60, we started to slow down our sexual life, then for the last three years preceding his death, we stopped our sexual activity completely. That was the only change in our retired life. We still slept together, ate together, volunteered at the same hospital and even played piano together. Two years ago we went on a "honeymoon" cruise, a trip that our children gave us on our anniversary.

Q: Do you miss sex?

A: Not necessarily. Sex united us during our adult life. Once we became united nothing could separate us; absence of sex, family problems, children leaving home, retirement, health problems, etc. Together we had a very happy life to the end.

Table 24 describes the sexual profile of old married people, both seniors, and still living together. Seniors cohabiting with a senior of the opposite sex without being married are not included. Within our total population of 2722 seniors, we located 250 couples that were married before retirement and both spouses are seniors. They were married well before they both became seniors. There were more than 250 married couples, but only in 250 of them were we able to interview husband and wife (always separately and never together). Of the 250 women that were interviewed, half of them were sexually active within the marriage confinement with varying degrees of sexual activity and varying degrees of love and emotional attachment. The other half had given up sex within the marital confinement. Among those who gave up, some of them claimed that it became painful due to vaginal atresia or narrowing, senile vaginitis, or vaginal irritation to sex. It should be specified that these women never sought medical help for this treatable disability. Others lost interest, or barely had any interest in it, and no longer considered a husband's request enough motivation to keep doing it. During their adult life they went along with sex to keep peace in the family, but now they no longer feel obligated to respect their husband's wishes. Other women gave it up because they wanted to participate fully in orgasm insisting on careful and elaborate preparation that the male partner refused to provide or did not know how to provide. Some women claimed that, although they were still interested in sex, the spouse could not participate because of physical handicap or impotence or because he did not want to have sex with them. Some women had a hidden dislike for their husbands and now it was in the open. These women refuse sex almost out of revenge for previously presumed abuses. Some women had no explanation and said they just gave it up. Some women tried to give us a religious or moral explanation, but on further questioning we found this to be more of an excuse than an explanation. Finally, some turned to outside affairs or masturbation.

I am now 73 years old, married to the same woman for 43 years. No children. My wife and I were school janitors until our retirement about twenty years ago. Nothing special about our sexual life except that as we aged I got more interested in sex and she lost more and more interest in it. Starting ten years ago, it looked like *she was doing to me a great favor each time she consented to sex. So about three years ago I started going with prostitutes. A friend of mine who was doing the same thing showed me how to go by it. I go about once a week. For the last year I go now to the same lady. The only problem is that my wife, who now took charge of the budget, is starting to wonder where $50 to $60 a week disappears. She does not suspect anything, but I have to keep saving pennies here and there and pretend to eat outside in order to keep affording this luxury.*

Among the 250 senior males that were still married, a similar number (about half) stayed sexually faithful within marriage and the other half gave up sex within the marriage confinement. Reasons for giving up sex were either a physical handicap or a general weakness and debilitation that prevented them from providing the physical strength necessary for sex. Some also claimed a weak erection or complete impotence. Refusal of the spouse to participate or no more attraction to the spouse were also frequent reasons. Finally, some turned to outside affairs or masturbation.

There were 19 males with wives younger than 55: these wives were not included in this study, There were six senior females with husbands younger than 55: these 6 husbands were not included in study. There were 42 couples with a physically or mentally handicapped partner (included in handicapped list if above 55).

In summary, of the 250 couples within our population who have been married before retirement, only half of them had a sexual life limited to the marriage confinement. That left us with 125 couples, 125 husbands and 125 wives, without sex within the marriage confinement. Table 24 presents the outside sexual activity in these couples.

Concern About Physical Appearance in Seniors

All our senior subjects were asked their impression about their physical appearance as a mature/old person, how they think it affects their sexuality and what, if anything, they are doing about it (Table 25).

I have been a traveling salesman all my life until I retired eleven years ago. I am now 81 years old and still a bachelor. All my working years I have been concerned about my outside appearance. I have to be clean shaven, a clean shirt, tie, suit, and shining shoes everyday. I had to pay high attention to my physical appearance especially during my last working years because I knew that old salemen are not popular with the boss, and I had to work only on strict commission. Of course, this neat appearance paid off, sexually speaking, up to my retirement. I did not have to work hard to score. Just by the way a woman talked to me or smiled at me I knew that all I had to do was invite her for dinner and the same night we ended up on the same bed. Surprisingly, my advancing age did not discourage women regardless of their age.

Now, thank God, I am retired. Instead of shaving every day I grew a moustache and a beard and I no longer color my hair. I wear blue jeans and sneakers all the time. And you know what? Indirect and direct propositions from women keep coming as soon as I say I am a bachelor and retired salesman. There is something bizarre about this combination that attracts women. Anyway, for the last two years I completely lost interest in womanizing. For the last three months I have been seeing the same woman and we are talking about living together. I do not know if it will work because, previously, I never stayed too long with the same woman.

On the senior male side, there appears to be a limited concern about physical appearance. Most of them are neatly dressed, take a shower daily or every other day, change socks and underwear daily, shave daily, use body lotions minimally, brush their teeth once or twice a day, and in general are concerned about a neat traditional appearance without excess of any kind. Body neglect was minimal in our group of 1239 senior males.

Some senior males, about one in four, showed excessive concern about physical appearance thinking that it would improve their sexual performance. Plastic surgery on different parts of the body, mostly liposuction on a pot belly, was rare (less than 1%), hair transplant in less than 1% of the cases, and surgical procedures such as baculum insertion on the penis or penis elongation were seen in a little more than 1%.

The intake of Viagra and/or herbal medications to improve different aspects of sexual performance such as sexual desire, extended duration of erection and ejaculation is becoming popular among senior men. This subject will be discussed in length in the next chapter. Some mention definite improvement with Viagra and the like, others a temporary one and some no result at all: 17.6% of senior males are currently using or have used these types of medication. Excessive attention to clothing, hair style, etc., in order to look younger and be more sexually attractive was evident in about 6% of the senior male population. Excessive concern and even hysteria against appearing old was expressed by 9.3% of senior males. Some senior males are sensitive about their age: 16.6% frankly lie about it and always shorten their real age by five to ten years, and 22.4% refuse to tell their age when asked about it.

What do I do about my physical appearance? Enough, but not excessively. My husband is 68 years and I am 66. He is good looking, even now, and has a way of talking to women and giving them compliments that make them blush and they keep looking at him embarrassingly. So I have to keep appearing as young and as beautiful as I can. I do not think he has ever been unfaithful, but you never know. As we advance in age, I am desperately finding that I have more and more women to compete with. Frankly, I am excessively jealous. I had plastic surgeries once on my face, once on my breasts, and once in the vagina. I do physical exercises and watch my diet to stay slim because I know he dislikes overweight women. I promptly comply to all his sexual requests although, between us, I will be satisfied with much less. I never put on excessive make-up or wear flashy clothing because I heard him making sarcastic comments in this matter. I know he loves me and will never hurt me, and sometimes I wonder if he is only teasing me with his outside appearance in order to keep me attracted to him. All in all, I consider that I have a happy senior life.

On the female side, the picture is completely different. About half of senior women limit themselves to a neat appearance and they neither overexpose their age, nor try to hide it. They have a classical appearance in their clothing, hair style, make-up. The other half of the senior women is a completely different story. They are convinced that youth and beauty go together, entirely and exclusively determine sexual attraction, and they overdo it in this matter. Plastic surgery is very popular among aging ladies: 7.5% had it once, and 3% more than once. Since the rejuvenating effect of plastic surgery lasts five years at most, the earlier in senior life it is performed, the more often it has to be repeated. The most popular procedures are on the abdomen (liposuction), on the breasts, on the face (eyelids), on the hips, and practically on every part of the body.

A popular procedure, although not well known is vaginal plastic. The senior lady complains of some urinary incontinence and a feeling of the womb dropping through the vagina. The gynecologist surgically lifts up or removes the uterus through the vagina and in the process he elongates and narrows the vaginal cavity. This, supposedly, markedly improves sexual activity for the two coital partners. This surgical procedure requires a skilled surgeon and its effects also last about five years. About 5% of women had such a procedure. It is now less popular because with less and less children per family and the practice of episiotomy (surgically opening the vaginal entrance for the passage of newborn, and repairing it after delivery), there is less damage to the vagina during childbirth and less need for surgical repair later in life. It is still frequently performed.

Viagra and other similar herb medications are not as popular, or rather are not advertised as much among women as they are among men. However, they are making their way and are now used by 8.7% of our senior female population.

Excessive attention to clothing, hair style, make-up is very popular and very expensive. About 39% of senior women indulge in it and overdo it. I use the word "overdo" when a senior woman spends more money on it than when she was young or adult. Concern about looking as old as they really are and trying to look much younger involves half of the senior women. A third of senior woman lie about their age and 80% of the others never tell their age.

In summary, only a small fraction of the senior men are concerned with their physical appearance and its relation to sexual attraction. The spreading use of Viagra is to be noted however. On the contrary, at least half of the senior women are concerned about looking younger with the belief that it will make them more attractive sexually: they overdo it, usually with limited success as will be seen later.

An Honest Look at Viagra and the Like

All the sexually active and inactive subjects were asked if they use or have used Viagra and/or similar drugs and what are their feelings about these drugs, regardless of whether they used them or not (Table 26).

Yes, I use Viagra frequently, and it saved my life, I mean my sexual life. I am now 81 years old and my wife is 18 years younger. We got married five years ago. It is my second marriage after my first wife died of leukemia about eight years ago. To my dismay, I was appalled to find out from the beginning of this marriage that my new wife wanted to be sexually active...almost every night. I could barely keep up with her. My erections were sometimes poor and not long lasting and I could sense her frustration and irritation. Am I to be made a cuckold by my gardener who appears to smile excessively at my wife and my wife responding likewise, as I could discretely see through the window curtain? There is no use firing the gardener because my wife is very social and easily approaches everybody. Is my marriage going to go on the rocks? I did not want to lose her because I became attached to her and I love her company. Then my doctor, with whom I shared my troubles, suggested Viagra. It was like magic. In the beginning I had some nausea and blurred vision when I took the pill, but my doctor suggested to take it at the end of a heavy meal. I never take Viagra more often than every third night, and the routine became very simple. We have a nice dinner outside with a glass of French red wine, I take the pill immediately after desert, and then we go home to bed. I have a hard and prolonged erection to the satisfaction of my wife. She appears to be contented with this regimen and no longer responds to the gardener's smiles.

The mechanism of male erection is very complex and still not completely understood. Sexual stimulation in men is cerebral in origin and is barely dependent on testosterone as it is in animals. It releases nitric oxide (NO) in the penis, which through an elaborate biochemical mechanism, increases blood flow in the penis, thus leading to erection: this involves the decrease of a specific enzyme, 5 (PDE5), and the increase of another, cGMP, in a mechanism still under study. Viagra increases the level of NO in the corpus cavernosum of the penis, therefore increasing blood flow, which then leads to erection. It is to be noted that the involved enzymes in the erection of the penis are only a little different from those in the heart, retina of the eye, and visceral and skeletal muscles: Viagra intake is therefore expected to have some effect also on these organs in addition to its effect on the penis. The only real contraindication to Viagra is a severe heart condition. Viagra is retained in the body for about four hours, then is eliminated mostly through the liver and much less through the kidneys. Seniors who usually have a minimal to moderate impairment of these two organs will therefore retain Viagra for more than four hours.

The use of drugs or herbs for sexual stimulation is as old as the history of mankind. Every period in history and every culture had and still has its own fad in this matter. The history of aphrodisiacs is humorous to say the least. It goes from old wives' tales to the royal courts. The consumption of bulls' testicles has been popular in Europe for centuries. Rhinoceros horn is still popular in Asia and Africa, either in powder form or as the handle of a dagger. Currently in the USA we prefer either the purified, properly researched and properly advertised products like Viagra, or the herbs mostly from South America, which may not be properly researched but are certainly and consistently advertised. Let us first concentrate on Viagra.

Among the seniors using sexual stimulation about half of them use Viagra, and the others are using other products either isolatedly or, most of the time, in combination. Most of these products have been directed toward curing different degrees of male impotence, rather than female frigidity, since female frigidity, in men's opinion, does not interfere with coitus. Most of these products however act supposedly on women as well as men, although some products supposedly act preferentially on men, others on women. First there are vitamins (B_3-E), amnioacids (L. arginine), metals such as Zinc. Then, there are the herbs mostly from South America: Epimediam extract, Tributus terrestris, Rehmania root, Damiana leaf, and Jujube. Some like Yohimbe bark, Saw Palmetto, and Peruvian Maca are recommended for men, while others are preferentially recommended for women such as Motherwort, Avena Sativa, Cordyceps, Lycium Berry, Ginkgo Biloba, Mexican Wild Yam, Siberian Ginseng, Muira Puama and Passion Flower. It should be noted that men stay away from these herbs used in South America by women, supposedly because they are feminizing. It should also be emphasized that, while Viagra is now the most popular because it has been thoroughly investigated and intensely advertized, there certainly are some South American herbs that are just as sexually stimulating. They just have not been paid enough attention to. For those people who are concerned with the connotation associated with Viagra, these herbal medicines are definitely indicated or at least worth a trial.

Only one of the three homosexuals and seven out of 222 masturbation group were using Viagra and will not be included in this special study. Table 26 concentrates on the attitude of heterosexual and the poorly sexual group and their attitudes. Not all our seniors were familiar with Viagra since for some of them it became popular after we interviewed them. Table 26 put together senior people using Viagra and/or sexually stimulating herbs: 218 senior men and 129 senior women use or have used Viagra and/or the like. Therefore only 347 out of the total investigated population are using these drugs (12.7%). We distinguish these senior users in three categories:

- The sexually orgasmic seniors who definitely attribute a noticeable improvement in their sexual life to Viagra/herbs: 75 (34.4%) senior males and 23 (17.8%) senior ladies.
- The poorly orgasmic and the non-orgasmic who attribute some improvement in their sexual life to these drugs: 61 (28%) senior males and 25 (19.4%) senior women.
- Those who saw limited or no improvement and have discontinued it: 82 (37.6%) senior men and 81 (62.8%) senior ladies.

Do I use Viagra? I tried it for a short while but it did not work for me. I am now 64 years old and my wife divorced me for all kinds of reasons, but the real reason was because I became progressively impotent after I developed diabetes. First I tried all kinds of herbal medication, then Viagra. All it did to me was give me chest pain and severe stomach cramps. My doctor ordered me to stop it immediately. I tried to live a sexless life with a lady companion. She was very understanding and willing to go along with it, but I was becoming sexually frustrated, frequently attempting and yet unable to have a decent erection. We separated still good friends, and she occasionally visits me, always willing to resume the relationship.

I continuously have sexual fantasies and I frequently have sexual dreams of the violent type. I take sedatives every night in order to fall asleep.

In summary, only about one senior in eight is using Viagra and the like for sexual stimulation, about one senior man in six and one senior woman in twelve. Among senior men, roughly one-third gets great success, one-third limited success, and one-third no result. Among senior women, roughly two-thirds get no success, and the other third is equally divided between great success and limited success. The statistical significance of these numbers is limited however because the majority of the senior population has not been exposed to or heard of these medications: when asked about the use of these drugs, most seniors stated that they did not know much about them and were afraid to use them.

There is more progress to come concerning these drugs. The progress in improving sexuality started only after scientists and lay people understood that androgens and estrogens are not **sexual** hormones but purely **reproductive** hormones. It is unbelievable how many researchers, physicians, and lay people still believe that the administration of androgens and estrogens will improve sexuality. Even advertising about any "herb medicine" still claims that these herbs contain androgens or estrogen-like products. Excessive intake of estrogen appears to be associated with breast cancer and excessive intake of androgen appears to be associated with cancer of the prostate and even liver. True researchers on sexuality have finally come to a few important conclusions: first, sexuality has nothing to do with androgen and estrogen which are reproductive hormones, not sexual hormones; second, that sexual arousal directly originates in the brain or is mediated through the brain after sensory (mostly cutaneous) stimulation; third, sexual arousal is due to increased blood circulation in the genital area (penis, testicle, vagina). These findings facilitated research in the field of sexual arousal. Viagra does nothing else but increase blood circulation to the penis, to the clitoris, and to the vagina. Other drugs that will increase blood flow in the genital area are being studied and will soon be available. Viagra has shortcomings: the onset of action is one hour after absorption and lasts only four hours. Besides, general flushing, stomach upset, headache, hazy vision and general aches are not rare. Most of all, it could make any heart condition worse. A new drug, Vardenafil (Bayer and Glaxo-Smith-Kline) can act a little sooner, last a little longer and has fewer side effects. Another new drug, Cialis by Lilly is acting much faster, lasts as much as a day and a half, but also has side effects. These last two drugs are available in Europe and soon will reach the USA.

Finally, future research is directed to act directly on the brain. The first one of these drugs, Uprima by Abbott Laboratories, is already available in Europe: you place a little tablet under the tongue and within 15 minutes you have sexual desire and erection.

The future of pharmacological sexuality is promising. As far as seniors are concerned, it appears that taboos concerning their sexuality will soon be lifted and they could approach it just the same as any other age, thanks to these promising drugs. The advantage of young and adult over seniors as far as sexual potency is concerned may become a thing of the past. Sexual impotence may be as treatable as, for instance, diabetes. We may be witnessing the beginning of an era where impotence and frigidity will no longer be a handicap to sexuality.

Health Problems in Senior Citizens and Effect on Sex

We consider here the health problems of the 2722 interviewed seniors who are in relative good health. The bulk of the seriously sick seniors were among those that were not interviewed: 674 of 3396 or 19.8% were not interviewed mostly because they were seriously sick (Table 5).

Both male and female seniors are concerned about their health which has become a constant worry for them. Its effect on their sexual life is becoming more and more an open matter. Would a disease interfere with sexual activity or would sexual activity interfere with their health? Major diseases commonly are seen in seniorhood and the most frequently involved organs and the most frequent diseases are as follows (Table 27):

Heart
lungs
joints
obesity
diabetes
hypertension
mental problems (dementia; Alzheimer's; Parkinson)
physical handicap due to cerebro-vascular accident
prostate condition for men and genital prolapse for women

Many seniors are completely healthy and can remain perfectly healthy at any age, from 55 to 90 and beyond. Some can be found perfectly healthy in every respect (*mens sana in corpore sano* = a healthy mind in a healthy body). They are not diabetic or hypertensive. They have had no previous heart attack and they breathe slowly and profoundly without any difficulty. They have little or no arthritis and their back is not arched. They do not suffer from osteoporosis. They take no medication except for some vitamins and other antiaging medication or occasional sedative for backache. Their medicine cabinet is not filled with many drugs. They walk perfectly erect at a normal pace without any walking aid and they easily jog one to two miles a day. They do physical exercises in their home or at a nearby club. They swim or play golf in the summer. Some ice skate or even ski in the winter. Their mind is very active. They are either working, only semi-retired from an important position, or they still run their business or at least supervise it. They follow the stock market closely. They play bridge in the evening a couple of times a week. Many of them have hobbies such as painting, sculpture, ceramics or they join an orchestra. They are very involved in the activities of their community. They watch very little television except for the news in the morning and the evening. They take vacations in the summer and/or in the winter, and sometimes in between.

The group with health concerns is just as numerous as the healthy and their number increases more and more as we move to the older group, until almost everyone is non-healthy as we reach the late eighties and the nineties. They present a large variety of pictures in the different degrees of their health conditions.

Some are obese. They have been overweight either all their life, or have been accumulating weight since their retirement. They struggle with diets constantly and always unsuccessfully. Many of them have a touch of diabetes or are frankly diabetic and taking medication for it.

Some are hypertensive and take medication for it. This medication, mostly diuretics, makes them desire to urinate more frequently and they have to go more often to the bathroom especially at night. Their hypertension is often associated with persistent headache, and they take sedatives during the day and even at night.

Some have a cardiac condition because they had a previous heart attack or because they have a family history of heart problems. Others suffer from a combined heart/lung condition or just pulmonary insufficiency with breathing difficulty.

Some, if not most, suffer from arthritis. It can be in the back from a slipped disc or arched back; in the cervical spine with inability to turn the head fully; in the hip or knee; or heel spur resulting in difficulty or inability to walk because of pain. The arthritis can also be in the shoulders or hands. These various arthritic conditions result in limited movement of the specific joint with painful limitation of the corresponding function. Some are arthritic all over the body with decreasing mobility; first, they need a cane or a more complex walking device; then, a wheelchair with difficulty or inability to stand up; then, finally, the subjects become bedridden, first in a limited degree then totally. Many arthritics do not wait for this end-stage to become a couch potato glued to the television a good part of the day and even night. Beginning of inactivity almost automatically leads to increasing weight, and more and more until total inactivity. In these cases death is near, although limited activity can prolong life for many years.

In the male, let us not forget the prostatic condition resulting in urinary frequency, and in the female, genital prolapse also results in urinary frequency among other complaints. These conditions can be easily corrected.

The largest group of non-healthy individuals is represented by the mentally sick. The major mental illnesses are Alzheimer's disease, Parkinson's disease, and senile dementia. Many of these diseases are latent and unrecognized especially at the earliest stages. There are many other forms of mental illness in senior citizens that are difficult to categorize; a touch of aggressiveness, stubbornness, constant vocalizations, forgetfulness, etc., that make social contacts difficult and embarrassing.

All the non-healthy seniors and even some healthy ones are on medication of some kind, sometimes up to 20 different medications per day. These medications can be very expensive, although many of them are without any real curative effect. All seniors are at the mercy of advertising by pharmaceutical companies and salesmen who constantly promise miracle cures for any senior ailment. Some daring salesmen will even go from door to door trying to engage seniors in some drug or medical equipment program at no cost since Medicare will pay for most of it. More often than not, medical care represents a major drain on the senior's budget.

There are two other medical conditions specific to seniors and difficult to categorize, but that are frequently encountered, namely general weakness and apathy.

General and progressive weakness affects almost every senior at the end of life, even if there is no major illness. Some individuals start to get tired early in senior life, others as they advance in age. It is very unusual to reach the age of 90 without some kind of general weakness, although I have met some people in their nineties that are physically and mentally alert.

Apathy exists in all ages. It is the opposite of workaholism. These seniors had a job they did not like but made a living out of it. When they retired their basic apathy comes to the surface and predominates. They sit on a chair all day long doing nothing, barely reading a newspaper or watching television. Their conversations are dull and they barely speak anyway. They have very limited physical activity. For them, retirement is the greatest opportunity to do what they wanted all their life, which is to do nothing. Some get involved with a minor disease or invent one and they spend the rest of their life taking care of it.

I repeat that the bulk of the seriously sick seniors were not among the interviewed ones (Table 5). In the interviewed seniors we were mostly concerned with the role played by their sickness in their sexuality.

It would be a mistake to imagine a direct relationship between disease(s) and sexual activity. Although there is a vague relationship, I have seen numerous exceptions of very healthy individuals who are impotent and several handicapped individuals with noticeable sexual activity. In terms of the effects of these different states of health on senior sexuality, let us specify that many of these diseases are treatable although others are less, especially mental diseases, no matter what pharmaceutical companies say. One can lose weight, although it is difficult. Diabetes can be well treated if the affected subject carefully follows diet restriction and takes medication. High blood pressure can be lowered to normal or near normal although with some side effects from the medication. Heart conditions require special medical care but with proper changes in living style, namely less stress, one learns to adapt to it. There are numerous medications to treat arthritis, in fact too many, and well advertised new ones appear constantly on the market. In fact, one can learn to cope with, or at least slow down, the harm of many physical deficiencies.

I am 79 years old, a widower for fifteen years. I had a heart attack immediately after my wife's death, but I recovered very well after I had a triple coronary bypass. I retired from my job to avoid any stress, I went on a strict diet to lose weight and I do moderate daily exercises. I am now suffering from generalized arthritis, but it is responding to sedatives and to glucosamine-chondroitin, although I occasionally use a walker. Finally, I suffer from an enlarged prostate which makes me urinate frequently. My urologist wants to remove my prostate but I do not want to because he said the operation may put an end to my sexual life. He was very surprised to learn that I would prefer to suffer the inconvenience of an enlarged prostate rather than give up sex. Indeed, in spite of all my ailments I have sex at least twice a week, sometimes more. I started living with a regular companion two years after my wife passed away. She can barely keep up with me, sexually speaking, and I do not hesitate to get involved in casual affairs here and there to supplement my sexual needs.

Q: Aren't you concerned that this excessive sexual life may interfer with your health?

A: On the contrary, it keeps me young and I forget my ailments.

Table 28 shows that when senior health is not seriously compromised and is well treated, it barely interferes with senior sexuality. Comparing seniors with health concerns to seniors without any health concerns, sexual activity (of all types) goes from 75.1% to 84.2% in males and from 42.8% to 44.3% in females. Health conditions, when mild to moderate and when well treated, barely interfere with senior sexuality. This is completely different from seriously sick seniors where sexuality is barely existent (Table 5). The difference is much smaller among senior women (1.5%) than among senior men (9.1%). It therefore appears that senior women take much better care of their ailments than senior men.

Periods of Sexual Abstention Among Seniors

I am 66 years old, married for the past 40 years to my wife who is two years younger. Our three children are now living on their own, although the oldest, married with four children, is in need of financial help. I am a traveling representative of an important computer company with divisions all over the world. I happen to be away from my wife weeks and months at the time. My wife does not mind because she is very involved with our three children and our eight grandchildren. I am very attached to my wife, but I cannot stay away from sex for more than a couple of weeks at one time. At home I am faithful to my wife and family, but abroad I have developed a steady relationship with a woman in each different country, notwithstanding an occasional variation here and there.

Q: Does you wife know about your extramarital activities?

A: I do not think so, but I don't know. When I am home, I sometimes receive strange phone calls from overseas that could make her wonder.

Q: Do you think that your wife may be unfaithful to you when you are away?

A: Certainly not, I hope not. It would reflect on her relationship with the children and grandchildren. Besides, her interest in sex is very moderate, at most. She is barely orgasmic, anyway, and I am always the one to make sexual advances.

Periods of sexual abstention are variable among seniors and between senior men and women. Sexual abstention can result from many causes: separation, divorce, sickness, widowhood, prolonged trip for one partner with the two partners remaining faithful to each other, and so on. Table 29 does not mention if the end of abstention is return to the previous sexual partner or a different partner, as any partner may return to sexual activities with the same or another partner. Table 29 lists periods of abstention only during the senior life and it concerns only sexually active individuals that abstain periodically.

I am now 79 years old. I divorced my first husband at the age of 35 and the second one at the age of 52. I have been single since the second divorce. I don't like to live alone, although my interest in sex is at most moderate. I tried to live with another woman but when I found out that she was interested in a lesbian relationship, I walked away. For the last twenty years I lived with three different men. The first relationship lasted three years, followed by two years of loneliness. The second lasted four years followed by three years when I stayed alone. Now I am living with the same man for the last seven years.

Q: During the years you were alone, did you feel deprived of sex?

A: Not really, but I felt deprived of companionship.

Q: Do you enjoy sex when you engage in it?

A: Sometimes. I want you to know that I have developed expertise in arousing a man sexually. My successive companions appreciated that.

Q: But, do you like to be aroused sexually?

A: At this time in my life I suppose I could do without it. But I learned the hard way that the only way to keep a relationship going on, is never to reject any sexual request. Fortunately or unfortunately men need sex more than women. This is true at any age, and also true in old age.

It is obvious that senior women can take periods of abstention that last much longer than senior men. The bulk of senior males can abstain only between three to six months, while the bulk of senior females can easily abstain for a year or more. We will discuss later the reasons for this lengthy abstention in senior women, but we already have mentioned two reasons: the first is that there are more senior women that are sexually available than senior men; the other reason is that women are more "choosy" in replacing a departed partner, while senior men have more choice and can easily turn to a prostitute for instance.

We have not been able to establish a statistical difference between adults and seniors in terms of duration of sexual abstention. From the reliable data we were able to gather, and comparing with the Kinsey Report, it appears that young and adult have much shorter periods of sexual abstention than seniors. Both senior males and females abstain for longer periods than the younger generation, with the senior female more than the senior male.

Evaluation of Coitus by Senior Men

You want to know my general impression about sex in the senior age? Well, it is great for senior men, and there are many reasons.

Years ago, as a single man, I always had to run after girls, approach them carefully, convince them, prepare them, seduce them, use condoms against pregnancy and/or STD. I am now 82, and since the age of 69, when my wife passed away, I do not have the sexual problems I had in my youth. I am not an old bachelor, I am a new bachelor. I remember with amusement the "boy-meets-girl" parties in my youth and compare them to the seniors' parties. Somehow when a senior man is available there is something in his physical appearance that immediately signals his availability. Available senior women find all kinds of excuses to approach him, and even all married women have a lady friend or lady friends in need of an available man. Anyway, I do not run after anybody. I just wait to be approached directly or indirectly. There is no hard-to-get game or cock-teasing games from senior women. When I invite a senior lady to dinner it is well understood that we both have sex in mind. I may let it go the first date out of decency, but if at the second date we do not end up in bed, there will be no third date. I do not waste my time trying to steal a kiss or touch the lady here, but not there. Very quickly, one of us invites the other to the bedroom. I do not spend my time trying to convince her or to push her for sex. If anything I am the one to slow down the sexual process because of a slow arousal, while my partner, aroused or not, is immediately ready for coitus. In other words, the preparation is limited. What I like in senior ladies is that they don't feel that you are committed to them because you had sex. No precaution to take to avoid pregnancy or fear of sexually transmitted disease (STD) because we seniors are always clean in the matter.

Q: Do you think that you take advantage of these ladies?

A: Listen, I did not run after them, I make my intentions very clear, and I do not promise anything beyond a dinner invitation. These are very adult people who know the score.
Q: Do you sometimes get attached to one lady, beyond sex?
A: Of course. The senior lady I am with now, we have been together for five months, and we are planning to live together, but neither one of us wants to get married. We want to keep our freedom.
Q: Suppose one of you does not like the other, what next?
A: Well this is a free country. Whoever wants to break the relationship is free to pack up and go. No divorce, no traumatic break-up, no lawyer. It's great.

Out of a total of 1239 senior men that were interviewed, 931 or 75.1% were heterosexually active. We analyzed in detail their general description and their different impressions about their sexual activity (Table 30). The majority of senior men (86.3%) prefer to limit themselves to one female partner. Even those who go with prostitutes prefer to go with the same one. There were only a dozen senior men, mostly in the group of young seniors between 55 and 65 years of age, who were playboys and who were doing it for "show" because most of them were poor sexual performers.

The elaborate courtship, so characteristic of the young and adult, is all gone in senior age. A senior male frequently expects the first date to end up with sex, or at most the second date, and it is rare that he will wait to a third date. Most of the seniors (75.9%) will get involved in a relationship only if, from the beginning, there is an understanding that sex is the immediate and essential part of a new relationship. In fact, lack of sexual proposition on first date could make the senior woman worry about male impotence.

Senior males no longer expect to be in charge of the preparation and stimulation that precedes coitus. They expect it to be equally shared and they even appreciate extensive touching (35.9%) over their body including hand-penis (51.6%) and even mouth-penis (11.2%) because quite a few have difficulty in reaching and maintaining erection. Very few are satisfied with sex play only, and when it happens it is because they are partially or totally impotent and they keep trying. Some complain of short duration of penetration (10.8%) because of almost immediate ejaculation. Other complaints are incomplete erection (21.7%), difficult or no ejaculation (22.6%), or performing coitus for the sake of the female partner because the senior male is really not interested (10.1%).

In general, however, two-thirds are satisfied with the duration of coitus, and most of them (84.5%) are satisfied with their sexual life, at least most of the time. About half of them make it a point to prolong coitus in order to wait for the female partner to reach orgasm. About one senior in five is generally frustrated in his sex life.

Senior Female Evaluation of Coitus

We are three ladies living together in the same apartment. Our ages: 69, 72, 75. Two are widows, one is divorced. We are all retired. One does some volunteer work in the village library, the second some part-time secretarial work, and the third keeps the house. We are having a great time. Yes, we are sexually active, occasionally, but our basic rule is very strict: no man should go beyond our living room and all sexual activities are to be held outside. Surprisingly, the most sexually active among us is the oldest who regularly spends the night outside on the average of twice a week; her boyfriend, or I should say her senior man friend, occasionally fixes up a date for the other two. Our life is great except for the relative shortage of men, who are harder and harder to come by. We easily learned to do without them. We love our lives the way it is, and none of us will move away to live permanently with a man. In fact one of us, the youngest, turned down such a proposition. We often talk about sex but not the way we used to when much younger. We are not obsessed with sex, we are not hysterical about getting married and keeping a male friend. We recognize that sex is more important to men, and we go along with it to maintain a relationship. We are not frigid, however, and when one of us reaches a sexual climax, it is our subject of conversation for the next day. As I keep saying to the other two, sex is now casual.

Out of 1483 senior women that were interviewed, 471 or 31.8% were heterosexually active. We analyzed in detail their general description and their different impressions of their sexual activity (Table 31).

Senior women would limit their sexual activity almost always to one sexual partner (96% of the cases). Rarely would a senior woman start an new affair without terminating the old one first. Only in a couple of cases did we encounter a woman with a regular sexual partner and an "affair" on the side. Very rarely also would a senior woman get involved in a one-night affair, like meeting someone in a party, have sex the same night after a few drinks and never see that person again: this is frequent only in the much younger age. A senior woman may get involved sexually on the first date, but it is usually a rational planning with the idea of the relationship lasting longer. Senior women get involved sexually when they are in the mood in 44% of the cases and insist on a good preparation in 49% of the cases. With a regular partner, they are indifferent to sex (28.3%), they are annoyed with it (31.8%), and find it painful in 13.2% of the cases. When desirous for orgasm (49%) they insist on a good preparation which includes general touching including the breasts (56.9%), finger-vagina contact or hetero-masturbation (43.5%), and even mouth-vagina (28.3%). They are barely interested in more elaborate sex play, only 22.1%. They complain that the sexual act is too short (35.2%), and they mention no orgasm or incomplete orgasm in 59.7% of the cases.

Occasional masturbation before coitus or after coitus in an attempt to reach coital or post-coital orgasm was mentioned in 42% of the cases.

However, they are satisfied with coitus in 65.6%, and reach orgasm in 40.3% of the cases.

Sexually active women are generally satisfied with their sexual life in 65.6% of the cases and look for mutual orgasm in 64.2% of the cases.

General frustration about their sexual life is expressed by 29.7% of them.

In summary, the scenario of men running after women, and the women playing hard to get, is over in senior age, notwithstanding some women and even some men desperately hanging onto the old scenario. Both senior genders make their sexual intentions clear from the beginning of a relationship. It is not unusual to see the senior woman initiating the relationship and the senior man running away from it. Senior men have the increasing problem of progressive impotence or just lack of interest in sex, as they do not want to be bothered and are looking for other interests in life. Senior women also lose interest in sex unless it is orgasmic or unless they have a personal interest in maintaining the relationship. Promiscuity (more than one sexual partner at the time), which has always been more limited in women than in men, is practically all gone in senior age. Presex play is markedly diminished to the despair of orgasmic senior women who insist on it. A prolonged sexual act, pleasurable in presex, sex, and postsex, is reduced at each level. Although about two-thirds of the sexually active seniors find satisfaction in it, the number of sexually frustrated seniors is increasing with age. As will be seen later, simple companionship without little or no sex is slowly replacing sex.

Motivation for Heterosexual Activity in Seniors

In the following table we explore the reasons that lead senior citizens to desire coitus. These questions are not naive because from the beginning of this research it became immediately obvious that the motivation that leads seniors toward sexual activity are sometimes similar but sometimes different from the motivation of younger ages. Table 32 lists the different factors that lead senior men and senior women to join a partner of the opposite sex for the purpose of coitus. The same 931 senior men and 471 senior women that have been listed as heterosexually active are again listed here. The reasons given for this activity were multiple and each subject gave many reasons; about 2 to 3 reasons are given by each subject.

Why do I still like to be sexually active? It is an urge or a habit I carried from my younger age, I guess. I am now 73 years old and I have been married to the same woman for the last fifty years. I still love her the same way I loved her at the beginning of our marriage. I cheated on her only a couple of times while she was pregnant and I do not feel proud about it. It is an old story. When I was young I had sex with her in order to prove that I loved her. But now she does not need that proof anymore. Although we still have sex once or twice a week, we are much more casual about it. I still say it is a biological urge because I feel restless when, for some reason, we abstain for a couple of weeks. Or maybe it is just a habit. My wife is still so jealous at our age and so suspicious that if I diminish my sexual requests in any way, she will immediately suspect that I am having an outside affair. I guess I still want to prove to her that I am still a man, the old way. My ego always feels inflated when after an elaborate preparation I manage to have her reach a sexual climax. I know I have accomplished something special because the following day she is completely different. It is great to be sexually active in old age.

Twice as many senior men (73.6%) than senior women (36.5%) talk about a "biological urge." It was hard to make seniors define biological urge. Senior men speak about erections, senior women speak about vaginal irritation or itching, and both of them have sexual dreams and fantasies. Some seniors (40.7% senior men and 27.6% senior women) state that sexual activity keeps them young. Sex as a habit carried from previous age is mentioned by 28.6% of senior men and 48.8% of women. Coitus to satisfy partner is mentioned much less by senior men (9.5%) than by senior women (36.6%). Finally, as much as two-thirds of senior women mention love for the sexual partner, and only 21.8% of senior men mention it. Quite a few had outside affairs and quite a few also visited prostitutes regularly. Some would prefer to be more sexually active, others less. Other special reasons were given only in isolated cases.

Why do I still have sex in spite of my old age? I tell you why. It is the only way to keep your husband with you. It is the only way to prevent any of these available women floating around from stealing your man. I am 74 years old, divorced my first husband at the age of 40, and got remarried to my present husband about 20 years ago. He is a couple of years younger than I am, and I was still beautiful when I remarried. Anyway, about three years ago I told my husband that I was not interested in sex anymore and I would like to slow down. He did not appear to object and our sex activity dropped down to about once a month. God, was I in for a shock when I found out that he was having a regular affair with my twin sister, who also has been divorced and never remarried! What infuriated me the most is that he joked about it by saying that, since it was with my identical twin, it stayed in the family and was not really cheating! Eventually I found how to settle the problem. I managed to figure out that his sex requirements are about twice a week, rarely three times. So now I request from him that much sex, so that there is nothing left for any outside affair.

Out of 1483 senior women, 471 or 31.8% were sexually active, one form or another. The reasons for sexual activity mentioned by these senior women were completely different from those given by the male counterpart. The biological urge was not often mentioned. A large segment among them felt that sex kept them young. Two-thirds mentioned real love for the partner. Other frequent reasons were to show off a sex partner, the need to satisfy the male partner although they would rather do without sex, and they kept it only as a habit from younger age. Some were 'kept' financially, some preferred more sex, others less and even did without it altogether. Surprisingly only a few mentioned the religious or moral obligation to satisfy the husband or partner. Looking for a male prostitute or changing partners was not frequent among women.

The conclusion of the review of sex motivation in seniors is that the biological urge is still dominant in senior men while senior women are less "urged" biologically speaking, they have sex by habit in half of the cases and mention love in two-thirds of the cases. As we will see later and as already shown in this table sex is more individualized in senior women than in senior men.

Reasons for Sexual Inactivity in Seniors

Among the various functions of the human body, the sexual function is elusive and associated with numerous problems that are not encountered with other body functions or other body organs. For instance, the cardiovascular system carries the function of blood circulation, the gastrointestinal system carries nutrition, the brain carries the mental and cerebral functions, etc., and usually all these functions are carried smoothly. On the contrary, the "function" of the sexual organs, and the "purpose" of sex are more difficult to define.

The reason for these difficulties is that the genital system, in men as well as in women, carries a double function, namely the reproductive function and the sexual function. The reproductive function is the same in all animals and humans, but the sexual function as such is unique to the human species and has been added as a new function to the human genital organs. Animals copulate solely for reproductive purposes. To put it differently, the genital organs are purely reproductive in animals and not associated with any pleasure or orgasm to speak of. There is no sexuality in animals, only reproduction, although this statement will raise numerous objections. While in humans, the genital organs are still reproductive, they have essentially become sexual, searching for pleasure, that culminates in orgasmic pleasure. Some religious, moral, and even medical authorities still see the genital organs in humans as solely reproductive organs, but the lay person, who knows very well that reproduction is most of the time out of their mind when they relate sexually, is very much aware that the genital organs are sexual organs and barely reproductive organs. The only concern of the young and adult when they indulge in sex is not how to reproduce but how to avoid reproduction. As long as reproduction and sexuality co-exist, one can be sexually active under the 'shadow' of reproduction and does not have to separate one from the other. But, when it comes to senior citizens, there is no doubt or controversy about the function of the genital organs. They are purely and solely sexual organs and nothing else since the reproductive function has completely ceased. Senior citizens who indulge in sexual activity indulge only in sex and not in reproduction or trying to avoid reproduction. That genital organs in seniors are purely sexual organs does not simplify the problem for seniors however. The senior has to recognize, to confess to himself or herself as well as to others that he/she is looking solely for pure pleasure and pure satisfaction. And this is where the problem lies. Sole pleasure in senior sex has been and still is condemned, to some degree at least, in many people's minds, including some seniors themselves. This inability to recognize senior sexuality as purely pleasurable, as an end to itself, is the source of sexual inhibition and conflict in seniors.

I am now 81 years old and the last time I got involved sexually with a woman was at the age of 50. Since then I gave up sex completely. I got married when I was 27 and divorced two years later without any children. I had a couple of relationships afterwards but none worked. It is not that I am impotent, since I still have occasional erections and I occasionally fantasize about sex. It is just that I find that relationships with women are very complicated. Especially now in my old age, women have been approaching me frequently and aggressively. Am I a problem or are they the problem? Sometimes I feel paranoid about what they want from me. They are old and they behave like they are young. They are not so beautiful and they behave like they are beauty contestants. I had a few dates with a woman about ten years younger, and it was my last attempt. On our first date she received me in her home and asked me to wait a few minutes for her to be ready. It took her more than one hour to put on some horrible make-up before she was ready. Although I could see from inside her apartment that she lived rather modestly, she insisted on dining at a very expensive restaurant, ordering some bizarre and expensive food that she did not even eat. The second time we went out she wanted to go to a mall for some shopping and made all kinds of direct and indirect allusions for me to buy her a gift. After that, there was no third date with her or with any other woman for that matter.

Out of a population of 1239 senior males, 257 subjects or 20.7% were not sexual. The reasons given for this abstention were multiple, variegated and are an expression of the confusion in the minds of seniors concerning their sexuality (Table 33). Among the senior males the most frequent reasons given for abstention were impotence and/or no interest in sex. Frequent also were hesitation, fear of getting involved, fear of not being able to perform, preference to remain alone, and previous bad experience. Inability to find the proper partner was not common among senior males. To be noted is the fact that religious, moral, or family objections were rare. Few mentioned the social status of being with a companion without sexually performing.

I tell you why I don't have dates anymore. For women of my age, 67, there are not many available men. The few that are worth anything have been grabbed by aggressive women as soon as they are available. I consider myself still good looking and, without any plastic surgery or excessive make-up, I could still be attractive to a man of any age. I can have a good conversation, I am an excellent cook, and I do not have any expensive taste. But I do not know how, or rather I do not want to make advances to anybody. At any rate, the few seniors that are still available are highly uninteresting.

They are obsessed with sex and rather direct about it. I am not frigid and I would prefer climax with a man rather than through masturbation, but I do not want the relation to be only sexual and I insist on a good companionship. Besides, I am not that obsessed with sex anyway.

This year I had a blind date arranged by a friend. This friend insisted that I should call him myself to propose a date because, she said, this is how things go today. But I refused. Anyway he called, insisted that I should pick him up because he does not drive, he said. When he received me in his apartment, he proposed a drink directly in his bedroom! I walked away.

I am slowly coming to the conclusion that I should make my own life rather than waiting for a man to make it for me.

The reasons for female abstention are different from the male ones. The dominant reasons are inability to find a sexual partner, interest in companionship without sex, looking mostly for a husband or companion to support them, and family objections. Also frequent reasons are fear of not being sexually attractive, looking for the social status of being with a companion rather than looking for sex, frigidity, no interest in sex, and preference to remain alone. Less frequent are previous bad experience, painful sex, hostile to sex, some religious or moral objections, and not wanting to be involved.

Disequilibrium in the Number of Available Partners

I now am 73 years old and I never had a chance to settle down in life. I barely finished high school, then I took odd jobs. At the age of twenty, I volunteered for the U.S. Armed Forces. Then there was the Korean War, then the Vietnam War. After discharge I got a government scholarship for training in some kind of technology job. I tried to learn the trade for almost two years, but I did not do that well. Anyway I had to give it up because the scholarship ran out. I took odd jobs here and there. Then I ran into trouble with the law. I spent seven years in jail for armed robbery. In view of my good record in the army and because it was my first and only offense, I was released on probation for good behavior after seven years in jail. I settled down somehow and I took a job as a janitor in a big factory. It was a boring job. I stayed there for eleven years, then I was offered early retirement because they were laying off workers. It was not a big pension but combined with social security I have a modest but decent income. Eight years ago I started living with a woman about my age and also with a modest income. In the beginning of our relationship we tried sex, but neither of us was that interested and we gave it up. We share the expenses. She takes care of the house and cooking and I do odd things around the house, and I help as much as I can. These last few years have been the most peaceful in my life. But you can see, there was never an opportunity to settle down and have a family.

There are more senior women than men (Table 34). In the studied population of 2722 there were 84 men for every 100 women. In the 55-59 years old age group the difference, although noticeable, was rather modest: 93 males for 100 females. Then the difference increases slowly to the end of the seventies: in the 75-79 year old age group there were 77 males for 100 females. But in the 80-84 year old age group there was almost 1 man for 2 women and after 85 it is 1 man for 3 women. This repartition in our studied population was similar to one reported by the U.S. Bureau of Statistics.

Even under careful questioning, it is sometimes difficult to make the difference between sexually inactive, i.e. not interested in sex on one side, and on the other side, sexually deprived, i.e., sexually interested but no partner. In Table 35 we combine both as being sexually available, i.e. no fixed companion or spouse. The number of sexually available women was much greater than men, far beyond the larger female population. The proportion of sexually available men was 257 out of 1239 seniors or 20.7%, and sexually available women were 836 out of 1483 seniors or 56.4%. About one senior man out of five was sexually available, while more than half the senior women were sexually available. On the average there is, in senior age, three times as many sexually available women than men, with the proportions varying from one over ten to one over two depending on the age.

I am a sixty year old woman. I think I am still attractive, well educated (I am a lawyer) and doing well financially. I am still single because the big problem in my life was that my expectations were always above reality. When I started dating, a lot of guys were approaching me, and I considered that giving a kiss to a boy was doing him a great favor. In my twenties, I had a few sexual affairs here and there but it was never with a man I would have serious plans with because I would never allow premarital sex with a potential husband. When I graduated from law school at the age of twenty eight and got a job, Mom (may she rest in peace) and I always thought that nobody was good enough for me. Then things started to go wrong. I slowly found out that lawyers are not always popular and female lawyers are repellent. A few guys told me that they would never marry a lawyer because, since half of marriages end up in divorce, they would automatically be losers. Male lawyers in my age range are married and there is something psychologically wrong with those who are not. Then, the only serious propositions I got were divorced, widowers, or married men looking for sexual affairs and making the vague promise of a future divorce which never comes. No matter how much I lowered my expectations, no decent proposition came anymore. You want to know the last proposition I got? The garage mechanic who takes care of my car and who is diabetic, and divorced with three children. We tried sex and he was not even good at it. I hate myself for all the opportunities I missed in my life. I could now be married, with a large family, and even a grandmother.

I keep thinking about a nice boy I met in college. We were really attracted to each other and it was with him that I lost my virginity. But he was not ambitious and just wanted to look for a job after college. Not enough for me at that time. I would do anything to meet him again but my attempts to trace him were unsuccessful. I am obsessed with him.

What is left now? I guess I will join the crowd of senior women hunting for the few available senior men still left. Wish me good luck.

* * *

There is always a marked disequilibrium in terms of available sexual partners. In the adult population from 18-55 years of age, male and female population is more or less equal in number (Table 21). This equality in adult population is equal only in appearance however. The reality is that men are less available than women although they appear to be equal in number, and this is so for many reasons. Men die more frequently of accidents at any age. They are exposed more frequently to physical hard work and are therefore more frequently 'worn out,' exposed to serious diseases, and so on. Men are more frequently incapacitated, temporarily or permanently, than women. Wars and military assignments even when not associated with war and casualties, withdraw young soldiers from the sexual population. Prisons are filled mostly by men. Most of all men, more than women, have a tendency to get married much later in life, if at all. The result of all these factors is that as the population ages, there are less and less sexually available men and more sexually available women. Starting from fifty years of age, there are noticeably less sexually available men than sexually available women. Then the differences increase rapidly with age, so that by the age of 80 there are twice as many women as men. This disparity is really greater than these numbers appear to show if one excludes married couples or couples cohabitating together. The number of available senior men is very small compared to available senior women. How senior women deal with this limited male availability, or rather how senior men deal with this great female influx will be investigated later on.

Relationship Between Love and Sex in Seniors

Do I love my wife? I have been married to her for fifty years. We have gone through everything together: a serious sickness for each one of us, one daughter who died of leukemia, two years without a job, a serious fire in our house with damages only partly covered by insurance, and so on. My wife always worked part-time all her life and we now are both retired. She always controlled everything, the house, the finances, even my clothing. I don't want you to think that she wears the pants in the house because I have my independent life, my hobbies, my weekly card game with the guys, and so on. I just have a limited interest in the things she controls, and she is a good organizer. I know I cannot do without her and the idea that she could die first and I would be left alone gives me palpitations and dreadful anxieties. I do not think I could survive her departure. You know what, I do not think she will survive either if I die first. She is too used to discussing everything with me and at night we watch the news together in bed. That she could be alone or that I could be alone in bed at night would be something that neither of us would ever endure. I guess, yes, we are in love.

Q: How is your sex life?

A: It is still there about once a week. It means a little more to me than to her, although in the time to come we will do without it. It is not essential anymore to our relationship.

We asked our senior citizenry if they are in love with their partner either spouse or companion. It was sometimes difficult to define a love relationship among seniors. It was mostly a situation where sex could be considered exclusively with the loved partner, and yet sex was not necessary to the love relationship. Should the two partners separate for any reason, the departed partner will be deeply missed and most likely not replaced. A total of 1070 seniors (Table 36) out of the studied population of 2722 subjects or 39.3% were considered to fall in that strict category of being in love. There were 405 senior men or 32.7% of the total male population that declared themselves in love. About half (48.4%) of them associated their love with frequent sexuality, about one-fourth (26.4%) associated their love with limited sexuality, and another fourth (25.2%) with no sexuality.

Yes, I am tremendously attached and I love the man I live with. I am now 56 years old and he is twenty-five years older. My husband was alcoholic and he got shot and killed in a gunfight twenty-five years ago. He left me desperate and destitute with three young children. I guess I would have ended up on welfare if it was not for the man I met one year after I became a widow. He was already an old bachelor I suppose, but he became the father of my children. He was kind but authoritative and helped me adequately raise my three children. One of them even finished college. Now we live alone. I love him and will never leave him. His relationship with my oldest child, my son Eugene, has always been distant. I guess Eugene always remembers his father fondly and forgets all the abuses. Eugene is now well established, married with two children, and he and his wife proposed I leave my companion and come to live with them. I would never do that. I cannot imagine how they could make such a proposition. We are very attached to each other. He would be devastated and I would not be able to stand myself.

Q: How is your sexual life?

A: Relatively good, considering our differences in age. Frankly, I need it and I always did. Once to twice a week, and I always reach climax, although he sometimes does not reach orgasm.

Q: Suppose he gets seriously handicapped with a serious

ailment such as cerebral hemorrhage, Alzheimer's disease or severe heart attack. Would you place him in a nursing home?

A: I will never do that. He has been with me during my difficult years, and if he becomes handicapped, it will be the opportunity to show him and myself how grateful I can be. Anyway, since we are not legally married, I do not have the authority to make any decision. He is so kind that he often approaches the subject with me. But I find these conversations very distressing and we do not get anywhere. I think he made a very detailed Will in this matter, the details of which I am not aware of. He vaguely alluded to the fact that I am his heir and I am allowed to make all appropriate decisions.

Q: Should your companion die before you, how do you see your future?

A: He and I have discussed this matter as a joke. If one of us dies, the surviving one will carry a mourning for a minimum of six months and a maximum of one year, then is mandatorily ordered by the deceased one to start a new life.

Q: You said that sex is important for you. Suppose he becomes unable to perform? Would you look for another sex partner?

A: Never. We have been faithful to each other from the beginning of our relationship. We love each other and I would never hurt him. I enjoy sex, but I do not consider it essential.

There were 665 senior females (or 44.8%) of the total female population who declared themselves in love. Of them, 26.9% associated their love with frequent sexuality, 19.8% with limited sexuality, and 53.2% with no sexuality at all.

The conclusion from these figures is that three-fourths of senior men (74.8%) consider sex an important aspect of their love, while a little less than half (46.7%) of the senior women do. Sex is more necessary for senior men's love than for senior women's love. It is true, however, that men easily confuse love and sex on one side, and, on the other, women easily declare themselves in love even without sexual involvement.

Sex Without Love for Sex Partner

My wife and I retired five years ago at the age of 65 the mandatory retirement age in the company where we have been working together. We have one daughter, who is married and lives in California. Since we retired, we are getting along more or less, she is trying to find an occupation of her interest and I am trying to find my own. There is no love lost between us, and we have what I would call a marriage of convenience where we share the expenses, and where we agree that to live separately would be more expensive for each one of us. We are together by habit, a strong habit that neither of us wants to break, or dares to break.

Q: How is your sexual life?

A: It has been OK during our working years. I had a few sexual affairs on the side during our working years. She might have done the same thing, although she is not as sexually oriented as I am. We both gave each other our hard work as an excuse for our rather limited sexual life, promising each other a new honeymoon when we retired. Well, we retired, and there was no honeymoon. With some insistence on my part and some reluctance on hers, we agreed to one sexual act a week. That's it.

Q: Do you feel that you love your wife when you have sex?

A: On the contrary. It is during sex that I realize that we do not love each other anymore.

Q: Have you considered sex with a different person than your wife?

A: Well I have a friend who visits prostitutes and he may take me along.

Table 37 lists the seniors engaging in sexual activity without any real love for the sexual partner. Again, sex in love means a senior individual conceives sex only with the loved person, while sex without love means that the senior individual would replace the sexual partner if they grow apart, or would carry two sexual affairs at the same time.

On the senior male side, 628 out of 931 sexually active individuals (67.5%) declare that there is no real love in their sexual relations. These non-loving senior males relate sexually to more or less four equal groups of female partners: spouses, 19%; regular companion, 15%; outside affairs, 23.3%; and prostitutes, 20.8%.

I am 62 years old and I met this man about two years ago. He is five years older, well to do, and in good health. He has been a widow for a couple of years and, the way I figured, he was looking for a sexual companion. On my side I had a modest income and did not mind somebody else paying part of my expenses. Therefore I fitted the bill. He barely needs anything else from me because we always eat out and a cleaning girl keeps his apartment neat. I do not play with words, so I plainly state that I am kept. He can be generous. For instance, I needed all my teeth done over and he paid the whole bill. But he can also be tight with money and will not buy me expensive jewelry for my birthday, regardless how much I allude to it.

Q: How is your sexual life?

A: He is very demanding, almost every night.

Q; Do you reach sexual climax?

A: Never. He is always precipitous in reaching orgasm. Besides, practically all my life, I did not reach a climax, not even through masturbation. I guess that during all my life I considered sex as a way to reach a man and nothing else.

Q: Do you love him?

A: Of course not. I never got attached to a man in my life. I consider it too dangerous, and I do not want to lose control.

Q: Does he love you?

A: He loves only himself. Besides, I do not want anybody to become strongly attached to me. It makes separation difficult.

Q: How do you envision the future of your relationship?

A: Not too long, unless he becomes less tight with money. It is OK now.

On the senior female side, 160 out of 471 sexually active individuals (34%) declare that there is no real love in their sexual relation. These non-loving senior females relate sexually to: spouses, 11.9%; regular companion, 18.7%; outside affairs, 3%; and only a couple of senior women used a male prostitute.

The conclusion is, among the sexually active, two-thirds of senior men and one-third of senior women are not in love. Senior men, as a sex substitute or sex addition, generously use outside affairs and/or prostitutes, while senior women stay away from them.

Sexually Active Seniors Wishing to Give Up Sex

In the process of investigating sexuality in the senior population and the factors leading them to sexual activity, we asked them who is markedly interested in sex, or on the contrary, who has little or no interest in it and does not mind giving it up because of little or no interest. Table 38 lists among the sexually active seniors those who would not mind retiring from sex, although still active in it.

I just reached eighty. My wife passed away eleven years ago and a year later I married her sister. I was not really looking for any sexual activity, I just wanted somebody to help me keep the house. As soon as my wife passed away, my sister-in-law, age 62, offered to help keep the house, do some shopping and cooking, help with the laundry, etc. At first she came twice a week, then more frequently, then every day, then longer and longer every day. Then her daughter came from Chicago especially to see me. She stated rather strongly that my relationship with her mother was irregular, subject to gossip and that we should get married. I did not see anything wrong with that although I made it clear that I had no sexual interest. But my sister-in-law had always been jealous of my wife. She insisted that we sleep in the same bed and that I should try Viagra. Well, we have sex about once a week, and a poor performance on my part, I should say. Anyway, she takes care of the sexual preparation and performs all the sexual motions. She gets on top of me, and I just lie passively on my back.

I like her company, and I am happy to live with her, but I would like to find a way to send her a strong message that I have no interest in sex. I tell her that repeatedly, but I guess she hears only what she wants to hear.

On the senior male side, only 48 out of 931 sexually active individuals (5.2%) would prefer to give it up. The distribution is irregularly spread within different age groups, but is higher in the eighties plus group.

On the female side, 101 out of 471 sexually active individuals (21.4%) would prefer to give up sex and it is more or less evenly distributed among the different ages even in the eighty plus group.

Needless to say all those who wanted to give up sex belong to the poorly or non-orgasmic group among senior males and to the non-climactic group among the senior females. We asked all these seniors who would give up sex the reasons why they kept being sexually active anyway. We found two types of answers more or less evenly distributed among them. Half of them answered that it was mostly at the request of the partner who was still interested in sex. The other half wanted to demonstrate to themselves and/or to the others, mostly to their sexual partner, that they were still capable of sexual activity.

It should be mentioned that this "giving up" group was not necessarily looking to interrupt the relationship. They just wish to interrupt the sexual aspect of it.

Importance of Companionship Among Seniors

How much is companionship, either in marriage or simple companionship without marriage, meaningful to senior citizens is a question we asked all sexually active seniors (Table 39). We specifically asked them to compare the importance of sexuality and companionship in their reciprocal relationship.

My wife and I are passed eighty and we are aging gracefully. We do everything together such as cleaning the house, shopping, cooking, laundry. Our best time is in bed at night when we watch television. We don't visit people and we do not need to. Our children and grandchildren visit us for Christmas and Thanksgiving. Lately my wife started to forget things. I guess it is common in our age, and I watch her carefully.

Q: How is your sexual life?

A; We started to slow down ten years ago and our last intercourse was two to three years ago.

Q: Do you miss sex?

A: Not really, we just forgot about it.

Q: Would your relationship change in any way if you were sexually active?

A: Absolutely not. Maybe early in our senior age we may have thought that our relationship would be compromised with diminishing sexual activity, but time proved that it is not so. We both are happier that we feel the same toward each other even without sex.

Among sexually active senior men, 27.1% declared that sex was more important than companionship, 32.9% just as important, 16.8% less important, 23.3% were hesitant about the answer.

I am 75 years old, and the man I am living with is a widower two years younger. We have been living together for the past eleven years. Is sex important in maintaining our relationship? It is hard to say. In the beginning of our relationship, the first year we met, sex was very important, at least more important to him than to me. With the passing years, however, as we became fond of each other and as we found more and more common interests, sex played less and less of a role in our relationship. We have not stopped completely, far from it. I remember in the beginning how he used to be angry when I refused his advances for whatever reason, or even when I was completely passive and indifferent during sex. Now he has calmed down and, when I say no, he completely forgets about it.

Sex, however, still plays an important role in our life: whenever we have a serious argument and we do not talk to each other for a day or two, sex always precedes, or is associated with, or immediately follows our reconciliation. I even wonder sometimes if he gets into an argument at the slightest reason just as a way for him to signal a sexual desire.

Q: Would your relation persist if your sexual activity is terminated?

A: Absolutely, it will stay as it is.

Among sexually active senior women, about half of them (48.4%) declared sex less important than companionship, 29.5% just as important, only 11.9% more important, and 10.2% were hesitant.

It should be recalled here from Table 19, that 721 out of 931 or 77.4% of sexually active senior men are orgasmic and 190 out of 471 or 40.3% of sexually active senior women are orgasmic. Therefore, although orgasmicity is meaningful for senior men as well as senior women, more senior men give priority to sex over companionship, while in senior women it is the opposite. However, 32.9% of senior men, and 29.5% of senior women think that both are equally important. Therefore, Table 39 shows that sexuality is not a serious factor of discord among senior citizens. This is so different from the young and adult group where sexual problems are an important factor for discord. Among senior citizens, good companionship, even with limited or no sex, is a rising factor in compatibility.

Examples of the Three Attitudes Among Seniors Regarding Sexuality

We have previously mentioned that senior citizens are faced with a dilemma when it comes to sexuality. This dilemma arises from the fact that hormonal stimulation and the function of procreation have disappeared in senior age, and seniors are left with how to account for their sexual desire, if any, in the absence of reproductive and hormonal function. The quandary concerning senior sexuality is great and one is tempted to take different and even opposite directions. In facing this dilemma, seniors may take three different approaches to which we have alluded previously and which will now be described in detail.

* * *

Case History of the First Approach, the Non-Sexual Group

I am a 68 year old woman. I have been a school teacher from the age of 20 to 60, when I took an early retirement. I have three daughters; two are married with their own children; the last one is a lesbian living with another woman.

I have never been really interested in sex. I started sex at the age of 24 when I married. I was neither repulsed or annoyed by it, I just considered it something you had to endure. My husband always made the first approach. In the beginning of our marriage my husband approached me two to three times a week. I always complied, although I never experienced orgasm. I knew what orgasm was only through what my sister and other friends told me, but I never experienced it. I enjoyed being pregnant because for me it was a period of rest from sex. After the age of 40, I started to make excuses for refusing sexual intercourse and by the age of 50, we stopped altogether. I suspect that my husband was having an affair with a colleague of mine, but I did not care. In fact, I welcomed it as it helped keep him away from me.

My husband and I are still married, both retired and living in the same apartment. We barely talk to each other except during meals and we each have separate rooms. We watch television in the evening, but most of the time he takes off his hearing aid and reads the newspaper. The only activity in the house is when our children and grandchildren visit and, very rarely, when we receive friends.

Q. In view of your early retirement from sexual activity, do you think you missed something in your life?

A. Not really. The real purpose of sex is to have children. Procreation is what nature made sex for. In the whole animal kingdom, animals copulate to reproduce. I had three children and I consider that sex fulfilled and terminated its function. To use sex for any other purpose is abnormal.

Q. You said that your sister and your friends had described sexual orgasm to you. Do you wish you could have experienced orgasm?

A. Not really; I am not sure. My sister mentioned that she would get angry at her husband when he did not go through what she called 'preparation', ejaculated quickly, and went to sleep. This had even been the source of arguments between them. My sister is three years younger than I am and she recently mentioned that she still occasionally experiences orgasm. Good for her, I am not interested. I do not want to get involved with that and I am happy with the way things are.

Q. Your three daughters, the two who are married and the lesbian, do they experience orgasms?

A. The first married one I do not know, but the other married one told me she does. My lesbian daughter mentioned during an argument about her homosexuality that she had tried heterosexuality but never experienced orgasms as she does with her lesbian partner. For me orgasm is too complicated

and I am glad I am not involved.
Q. If you had experienced sexual orgasm would you have been more compliant with your husband's requests, and in this case would your marriage have been happier?
A. I am happy the way my marriage has been and is now going. I do not want to take any chance by changing things.
Q. Has your husband made sexual requests lately?
A. Not for the last ten years.
Q. Do you think you have deprived your husband of something during your married life?
A. I gave him what I was able to give. Although I was a working mother, I raised my family adequately. I kept a nice home, and my husband considered himself happy in it. At least, that is what he says.
Q. Do you have sexual fantasies?
A. I used to, but no more.
Q. Any sexual dreams?
A. Occasionally. Mostly nightmares associated with rape and other sexual brutalities.
Q. Did you ever wish to have an extramarital affair?
A. I had fantasies about it, but not lately.
Q. Do you have any questions?
A. Yes, I wonder how other couples of similar age behave sexually.

Some may give up sex altogether and form what I call the non-sexual group. Their physical strength may or may not start to decline and they may give it up suddenly or progressively, totally or almost totally. They see no sense, or any meaning in it, and may find relief in this new abstention. This is true mostly for those women who have not or barely have known orgasm and for whom sex was a duty and an important element of family harmony. The vaginal hygiene imposed by sex and menstruation was terminated with relief. They found emotional support in getting involved in the life of their children and grandchildren by providing baby sitting and needed financial support although sometimes their continuous presence may invade their children's privacy. They do not have to appear sexy anymore, be sexually seductive and attractive in terms of their clothing, wear painful high-heel shoes, use make-up, or maintain hair styles and pedicures/manicures. They worry about their general appearance in a more relaxed way. A sexless life with all the advantages that go with it becomes attractive and these senior women indulge in it. They now find male companionship rather boring with their continuous preoccupation with sex, and would prefer to join other women with the same thinking in different social clubs such as bridge, visiting museums, touring, or simply taking tea together and gossiping all day long. Some other women would rather stay alone, involved in some minimal activity such as reading, watching TV, visiting children or grandchildren or other family relatives.

Some senior men also withdraw from sexuality and now feel threatened by the open advances of some senior women. The race for the few available senior men by the increasing number of senior women can become awful and reach clownish proportions. Some senior men enjoy being chased but most of them are annoyed by it and try to avoid it. They join men's clubs where they enjoy their own activities such as bridge, golf, fishing, physical education, etc. Many of these clubs are for 'men only.'

Some seniors may adopt a slightly negative attitude toward sex at the start of senior life, and this negativity increases more and more as they age. It is unbelievable how males and females separate themselves from each other and barely meet in their various social activities. They may still appear to form a harmonious couple in their private life but they have different social activities that completely ignore each other. In the matter of living alone without the opposite sex, women alone do much better than men alone. They manage to organize their lonely life without feeling much loneliness. They enjoy much more than men visiting children and grandchildren, or being with other women. On the contrary, men are bored with all these things and even with the company of other men. For one thing, women know how to keep the house clean, how to cook, how to shop at the supermarket, go to the cleaners, and so on. Men do not know any of these things and it is frequently hard to learn. They end up hiring a housekeeper and always eat out. A man needs the company of a woman, much more than a woman needs the company of a man. In general, the social life in which the women organize themselves has more variety and more life than the corresponding one organized by senior men. This asexual life may be the result of some social, moral, religious or family pressure, or at least it appears that way. The first and easiest way is to either give up sex altogether or to practice it in a discreetly hidden, unspoken way. This is very easy to do and it is done by many seniors. The pressures to be asexual or to be very discreet about it are tremendous. There is family pressure by children and other relatives who do not conceive sex in old age. There are religious considerations for those who see sex only as a reproductive function. There are moral considerations, which are similar to religious ones. Finally, there are social pressures which strongly condemn, criticize, and very often make ridiculous remarks and jokes about senior sex. Needless to say, all these pressures are directed more toward senior females and much less toward senior males who are often more or less excused for it.

What has been described here may approximately represent

one-fourth of the new life of the senior citizens.

Case History of the Second Approach, The Pretend Group

Mrs. DiMarco is a 72-year-old lady that my wife and I have known for many years and, although we are not close to her, we met her on numerous social occasions. Whenever we meet her socially, the scenario is almost routine: she will join a group of four or five people talking together, gets involved in the conversation, very quickly takes a central role in the conversation, then turns the subject of the conversation to everything concerning her: her big house, her children, her last vacation trip with her male companion, her recent shopping, and so on. Very slowly everybody leaves the group and when left alone she goes to join another group and starts all over. She divorced about 24 years ago, and now all her three children are grown up and gone, and she lives alone in a big house. She has always been average looking, not a great beauty, but the amount of make-up she uses has increased over the years. She always dresses like a teenager, and frequently brags that she and her youngest daughter still exchange clothes. The dresses she wears always stop above the knee, exposing extensively her legs covered with wrinkles and brown spots. My wife assured me that she is on her third facelift, and that she is planning another one. Any lady going to the beauty parlor has a great chance of meeting her there, because she goes there at least twice a week, and the busy beautician is working elaborately on the few hairs she has left, most likely destroying them with chemicals because she insists on red hair to hide all her white hair. Her nail polish is of the Korean type and very elaborate in its design. Her toe nails are sparkling red. Whenever she appears at a party she always is with a male companion whom she introduces as a friend but I suspect she is using an escort service, at least occasionally, because the companion is rarely the same. She is an addict to massage parlors, health spas and always brags about going on cruises with a companion. She tells other women that sex is no problem for her because she says she is never short of suitors. As long as I remember her she has always been 52 years old and she keeps mentioning it either directly or through indirect sentences such as: "In 1982, when I was 35 years old, we went on a cruise" thus giving listeners an opportunity to calculate her age. Her oldest daughter, whom she does not get along with, claims that she and her mother are the "same age." I happen to know her real age because a friend of hers who went to elementary school with her and who is now 72, told us about it. I could go on and on, enumerating in detail how Mrs. DiMarco is acting like a much younger person.

Mrs. DiMarco's behavior reminded me of a quotation in The Grapes of Wrath by John Steinbeck (Penguin Books, 1986. Paperback p. 199). "Ladies about whom revolve a thousand accouterments, ointments to grease themselves, coloring matters in vials—black, pink, red, white, green, silver—to change the color of hair, eyes, lips, nails, brows, lashes, lids...A bag of bottles, syringes, pills, powders, fluids, jellies to make their sexual intercourse safe, odorless, unproductive. And this apart from clothes. What a hell of a nuisance!...Disliking sun, and wind, and earth, resenting food and weariness, hating time that rarely makes them beautiful and always makes them old...[they are] thinking how the sun will dry [their] skin."

In summary, we have here a lady who absolutely refuses to face the fact that she has stepped into senior age. For her, senior age is absence of life, and if and when you are a senior you are stepping into a predeath condition. She does not conceive any kind of life in senior life and for her only adult activities are living activities and she has remained frozen in adult age.

This is another category of senior citizenry that may take what I will call the pretend attitude. The senior men refuse to acknowledge that something has changed when they get older. They want to pretend that they are still young and virile by behaving sexually the way they behaved in adult life. Between themselves senior men continuously talk about sex. They maintain their active sexuality through all kinds of techniques, such as a baculum insertion to maintain a rigid erection and recently by taking Viagra. They also believe in all kinds of advertising that promise a better sexual life and are regular adepts of all the stimulating herbs. It is fortunate that all these techniques are, if not effective, at least not harmful. They join health clubs and get involved in excessive physical exercises to improve their physical appearance in the belief that it will lead to a better sexual life. They often get remarried or involved with a younger companion in the belief that she will be sexually more stimulating. Unfortunately they often end up with limited sexual performances, thus increasing their frustration and also the frustration of the younger partner who was expecting more sex.

Some senior women also play a similar game–their own way. They never tell anyone their real age. They use excessive make-up, wear flashy clothing, and spend a fortune at the beauty parlor on their hair and finger and toe nails. It is not that they are so much interested in sex, but they maintain the appearance of being still sexually attractive the young way. Most if not all of them had plastic surgery on their face, breasts, and the rest of their body including vaginal surgery to reestablish the depth and the narrowness of their vagina. They frequently go to health spas. The rejuvenating effect of plastic surgery is almost never long lasting and it has to be repeated every few years. Liposuction on every part of the body is definitely preferred to dieting. This behavior can be so excessive that it becomes embarrassing to the family, mostly the children. Sometimes it takes the aspect of financial irresponsibility when the senior woman gets involved with a younger man and has lied about her age in the belief that plastic surgery has rejuvenated her. If we compare senior men and women in this respect, I would say that men lie about age much less frequently and most of the time keep a certain element of rationality when involved with a younger female partner. When a senior woman becomes involved with a younger man, which is much less frequent, she can become erratic and financially irresponsible, thus leading the children, and future heirs, to take legal action. It is true, however, that in this matter society and the law are much more tolerant of senior men than of senior women.

This second attitude is to keep going for it–the adult way, i.e., the way it was before the age of 55. These men and women conceive sex the way they practiced it in earlier age, do not conceive it differently, and keep hanging on to it for as long as possible.

This second type of senior life involves another fourth of the senior citizenry.

Case History of the Third Approach, The Progressive Group

Mrs. Thompson was 58 years old when I met her for the first time. She came to see me for a regular check-up and also because her previous gynecologist has put her on Hormone Replacement Therapy or HRT with a small dose of estrogen (Premarin 0.625mg twice a day). She wanted to give it up permanently and in fact she has stopped taking it for the last month and wanted my advice about it. She presented no symptoms of estrogen withdrawal such as hot flashes and in fact she felt much calmer and slept better since she stopped estrogen therapy. I agreed with her that she should not resume it and suggested instead a healthy diet and daily exercise. Her husband had died of cerebral hemorrhage eight months ago and since she had some difficulty in falling asleep, I recommended a herbal infusion of Chamomile to be taken at bedtime. She appeared generally depressed since her recent widowhood and was rather bored in not knowing what to do with all her free time. She has three sons all married with their own children and although her daughters-in-law were polite with her, she did not feel welcome by them. She limits her visits to occasional babysitting, to birthdays and anniversaries. She only had one real friend, a girlfriend from childhood but she moved away. In conclusion she appeared to me as a typical lonely senior woman who, like so many others, will go on living for many decades because they will take good care of their health, but continuously preoccupied and unoccupied. I did not recommend any antidepressant because she did not ask for it and I did not see the need of it. I suggested a return visit in six months.

I saw her nine months later. What a difference! It looked like it was not the same person anymore. Dynamic life was sparkling out of her body and out of any gesture she made or any word she pronounced! She did not wear any excessive make-up or fancy jewelry or flashy clothing. She immediately assured me that she did not have any plastic surgery. She was so full of life that I was short of words in describing her. She started talking or rather gushing so much that I could hardly keep up with her while taking notes. After having "enjoyed her depression" (these were her own words), she decided that she had enough pitying herself and took a job as an assistant buyer in a big department store, in the toy department. She did so well that within three months she was promoted to full buyer. She loved the job because she found it stimulating and she always recommended the proper toys that sold rather quickly. Although she had freedom of her own schedule, she found it too time consuming and recently switched to a three-day a week schedule: the store kept her anyway with a raise because she was doing the job just as effectively as in a full time schedule. She has been promised high level managerial position in the future if interested. She is not sure. She joined a sports club and does forty-five minutes of daily exercise religously, weekdays as well as weekends, in the sport club or at home. She learned bridge and now plays it with a group of interesting people once or twice a week. She goes to the theater once a month and joined art groups visiting museums once a month with the proper guide. She loves reading, not the "best sellers," but the classical masters such as Shakespeare and Hemingway and regularly reads for one hour every evening before going to sleep. Most of all she discovered or rather rediscovered sculpture. She had always been interested in it from her teens and all her life she was making plans to go back to it, but one way or another she kept postponing it. Now she decided to jump on it all the way: she joined a sculpture class once a week, then twice a week, and is planning for three times a week. She is now opening a small sculpture workshop in her garage. She quoted the prophet Hillel: "If I do not do it myself, who will do it for me, and if I do not do it now, when am I going to do it?" Well, she said, she is doing it all by herself and right now.

By herself, she approached the subject of sexuality without waiting for me to bring it up. Yes, she has a companion for the last six months. They have become very attached to each other, but they do not live together. She sees him about twice a week and he stays over in her place or she stays over in his place overnight once a week. Next month they may go on a cruise together. She hopes the relationship will last but he wants to get married and she absolutely does not want to, at least for the time being. She feels that with her busy life there is no room for a husband. Does she reach climax, I asked. Almost always because he is patient, clever, caring and he will not (and she would not) conceive coitus without orgasm either together or one after the other. I asked her which was the most important for her, her sexual life or sculpture, and whether the time spent with her companion interfered with sculpture or vice-versa. Her answer was strange and left me pondering. "They reinforce each other, she said. They are not separable and in fact they are the same thing. The day following a sexual climax, I am very creative in my sculpture: and in the night following a day of creative sculpture, I feel very amorous: a China syndrome."

How about her children, I asked. She does not visit them anymore and told them she is not the babysitting type; but they are welcome to visit her providing it is on a prearranged schedule. Her three children and their family visit her now about once a month on a rotation basis. They now all look forward to visiting her because she has mastered the art of selecting gifts for each one of them: her daughters-in-law always wear the clothing or jewelry she buys for them and now they use her as a confidante for their most intimate problems. Her grandchildren are all anxiously waiting for her gifts which she learned to dispense in relation to their school achievements.

There is a third attitude. A completely new approach to senior sexuality needs to be made, along with a "tabula rasa" of any previous consideration.

This third group of seniors neither gives up sexuality like the first group, nor pretend to ignore the existence of senior age like the second group. They form what I call the **progressive** group. Of course, when people do not know how to deal with a problem, the easy way out is either to refuse to deal with it or to continue to ignore it, as did the first two groups. A better way is to face it and deal with it, as does this third group. Every aspect of senior life is to be redefined, reshaped, made over, most of all enjoyed, and this includes senior sexuality. These progressive senior people are free to be sexually active if they want or do without it if they don't. But neither of these two attitudes is to be dictated by or copied from any younger age group. These new seniors are willing to face senior sexuality for what it is, what it should be, and what it could be. True, sexuality is not hormonal nor reproductive. These seniors consider sexuality an expression of personal enjoyment, as a combined enjoyment. It also is a mode of consecrating a relation between two people who want to be together rather than to stay alone. But sex, although sometimes a tremendous stimulant, is not always necessary to consolidate the relationship. This happy and harmonious goal may appear to be too ambitious but it is simple to reach if the seniors put aside any preconceived idea about sex in advanced age.

Some seniors, mostly those who have been previously orgasmic in their sexuality, decide to remain sexual, completely disregarding any concepts or pseudo concepts of social, moral, religious, or familial origin. The senior man chose to remain sexually orgasmic and, in this point of view, he completely ignored the presence of senior age at least in the beginning. They slowed down very progressively with old age, mostly because male sexuality requires physical effort and they were less and less capable of it.

The case of senior women is even more instructive (Table 40): 203 women were orgasmic just before the age of 55, and among them 161 remained orgasmic after age 55 (not necessarily with the same partner), while 42 gave up heterosexual orgasms for reasons such as widowhood, divorce, separation, or other reasons. Most of these 42 women recovered their orgasms through masturbation. But the astounding fact is that 29 senior women discovered orgasm only at senior age, 22 of them with a new sex partner. The impression given by these data is that for progressive seniors, sex, mostly orgasmic sex, is here to stay. They consider it a part of their new life and deny anyone the right to judge them. Women, specifically, hang on to orgasmic sexuality regardless of age and quite a few even discovered orgasm in old age.

The last point I want to make is that among progressive seniors the interrelationship between them is being revised. It is no longer the man who plays the role of the macho protector, the provider, the boss; or the woman who is charming, seductive, passive or submissive. These old concepts may have been necessary in the previous concepts of the family unit, but in senior relationships these differences and inequalities disappear. The role of each gender, and the interrelationship between them is revised and reconsidered. Specifically, women making the first approach and gesture is not uncommon.

The progressive group also forms one-fourth of the senior citizenry.

For analytic purposes the seniors had to be divided into three sharply different categories. Really, these are only three tendencies, rather than sharply delineated categories. Although the majority of seniors (about 75%) fall into one of the above three categories, there really is a fourth category of seniors (about 25%), who fall between the previous categories and whose behavior borrows various elements from each one. In some respects they belong to one category, and in other respects to a different one. They are sometimes hard to define.

In summary, in terms of sexuality, some seniors give it up, some try to keep it the old way, some try to discover a new way suitable to their new life, and finally others fall in between.

Matching Sexuality and General Activity

Different Sexualities: As mentioned in previous tables, sexuality in senior citizens presents a tremendous variety in quality and quantity regardless of age. For instance, one could meet a 60-year-old subject who is completely non-sexual, or an 85-year-old subject who is orgasmic twice a week. The only requirements for sexual activity in seniors are good health and an available sex partner although many healthy seniors with available partners may be sexless. What makes a senior subject sexually active or sexually inactive? Rather, what characterizes the general life of a sexually active senior as opposed to a sexually inactive one? The first step was to grade sexual activity. After trial and error, it was found best to divide the senior subjects into four categories, from the sexual point of view.

Category 1 is composed of those individuals who are orgasmic, i.e., who, at least once a week reach orgasm or climax during sexual intercourse, viz. ejaculation after adequate thrusts in male and satisfactory climax in female.

Category 2 is composed of individuals who practice masturbation and manage through this practice to reach ejaculation in male or climax in females.

Category 3 is composed of heterosexuals with poor sexual quality. It includes men with poor erection or limited or no ejaculation and women who are sexually passive.

Category 4 is also easy to define. It is composed of individuals who have no sex of any kind, neither heterosexual, homosexual, nor masturbation.

Although there were a few borderline cases that were studied individually, all the investigated seniors were placed in one of these four sexual categories.

There were only three homosexuals (all three senior males) in the study, all of them in the 55-59 age range and in view of their small number, they were not included in any statistical study. We ended with a classification shown in Table 41.

Different General Activities. In the next step, the general life of these senior citizens was investigated in their daily and weekly schedules. We recorded their jobs, their hobbies, their leisure time, their daily routines, and called this their general activity. These various aspects of senior life in general were carefully analyzed in an attempt to recognize among them groups with patterns of similar activities. After numerous searches we recognized four types of general activities that could characterize the life of these senior citizens, as follows (Table 42).

A. Hyperactivity. These subjects were and still are workaholics in advanced age. In spite of any partial or total retirement, they kept working excessively. It is usually their previous jobs which they never gave up. If they retired from their previous jobs, they took up a hobby in a very compulsive or excessive manner, such as playing golf or bridge all day long, or excessive sports exercise, or continuously watching the stock market. This hyperactivity, mostly associated with sports, may interfere with everything in life. They have a very busy schedule. We will call them hyperactive.

B. Creative activity. It is the best activity later in life. These subjects do what they want or rather what they always wanted to do all their lives but never had the time for it as they were busy making a living in a job they did not necessarily like. But now they devote themselves to the activity of their dreams such as music, sculpture, painting, traveling, writing, finances, etc. These people do not have to belong to high class society. Some of them are very creative in helping retarded children, or children with learning disabilities, or all kinds of disabled people. They are often volunteers in libraries or hospitals. Although they have a full schedule, they have time for relaxation. We will call them creative.

C. Moderate activity. These people may still be involved in their usual job, at least part-time. If retired they take up relaxing hobbies, but not excessively. A couple of times a week for instance they do volunteer work, play bridge, golf, go fishing. They may become involved in cooking, house cleaning, gardening, etc., and although moderately busy, they have enough free time. We will call them moderately active.

D. Inactivity. These people have completely retired and sometimes took early retirement. They are inactive and bored, or their activity is pointless. They may gain weight. They are "couch potatoes" watching TV, reading newspapers, or just sitting all day long. They have time for everything and they do nothing. We will call them inactive.

The categorization of our studied population (2719 subjects) into one of the above four general activities (A,B,C, D) was rather easy (Table 42), although it was sometimes difficult to decide whether an individual was hyperactive from Group A, or creative from Group B. This was decided on a case-by-case basis.

The problem we were faced with was how to match the four different categories of sexualities (orgasmic 1, masturbation 2, poor sexuality 3, or no sex 4) with the four different types of general activities (hyperactive A, creative B, moderately active C, or inactive D). The purpose of this matching was to determine if there was any relationship between the different categories of sexual activities and the different types of general activity.

The male population (N=1236) is presented in Tables 43 and 44, and the female population (N=1483) in Tables 45 and 46. In each of these four tables, each investigated population is presented into age groups five years apart from 55 to 85+ years of age the same way it was presented in previous tables. In Tables 43 and 45, the population is divided into four segments representing the four types of general activities (A,B,C,D) and each segment is divided into four sub-segments each representing the four categories of sexualities (1,2,3,4). In Tables 44 and 46, the same population is divided into four segments representing the four types of sexualities 1,2,3,4, and each segment is divided into four sub-segments each representing the four categories of general activities A,B,C,D. This double presentation is not redundant: Tables 43 and 45 show how men and women with different general activities behave sexually; Tables 44 and 46 show how people with different sexualities behave in general. These two opposite points of view are really complementary. Each segment of the population could accurately be identified in terms of sexual activity, general activity, and the relation between both.

These four tables (43 to 46) exhibit the most important features of senior sexuality and summarize the essential findings of this research. It is necessary for the reader to become familiar with them. Many impressions are elicited from these tables and diagrams and significant conclusions can be drawn from them.

Table 43, Activity A, shows that out of 266 hyperactive male subjects, 71 percent are orgasmic, 17.7 percent attempt to be orgasmic, while masturbation and no sexuality are negligible (6.8 and 4.5 percent respectively). This is even more obvious with the 469 "creative" male subjects (Activity B of Table 43): 84.4%

are orgasmic, while the other three categories of sexualities are negligible: 4.3, 8.3 and 3.0% respectively. Out of 233 moderately active men (Activity C of Table 43) 54.9% are orgasmic, 24% attempt to be, while 3.5% masturbate, and 17.6% are non sexual. When it comes to the 268 inactive men (Category D of Table 43) only 3% are orgasmic, 25.4% attempt to be, masturbation is negligible, and the bulk, 70.9%, are non-sexual. Table 43 therefore demonstrates that hyperactive/creative senior males are sexually active and orgasmic, and generally inactive seniors are sexually inactive. This is even more striking with creativity alone which shows the highest percentage of orgasm (84.4%) and the lowest percentage (3.0%) of non-sexuality.

Is the reverse true, i.e., are most orgasmic men hyperactive-creative? This is demonstrated in Table 44. Out of 721 orgasmic men (Category 1), 26.2% are hyperactive, 54.9% are creative, 17.8% are moderately active and only 1.1% are inactive. Orgasm through masturbation (Category 2) shows almost the same results as orgasm through heterosexuality (Category 1). Poor heterosexuality (Category 3) shows an almost equal distribution between the various activities. Out of 257 non-sexual men (Category 4), the bulk of them (73.9%) are "couch potatoes."

The conclusion from Tables 43 and 44 is that the great majority of hyperactive men and even more so of creative men are orgasmic, while the majority of inactive men are non-sexual. And reversely, the great majority of orgasmic men are hyperactive and even more so are creative, while the majority of non-sexual men are inactive. It is to be noted that poor sexuality occupies an intermediate position among the different activities. To be noted also is that orgasm through masturbation is associated with the same high level of hyperactivity/creativity as orgasm through heterosexuality, although this series (N=48) is rather small to draw any conclusions.

Let us now look at the women's side. The series is impressive in number and valuable conclusions can be drawn. The remarks are similar to those presented in men. In the female population (N=1483), it is also obvious that hyperactivity-creativity on one side and orgasmicity on the other side go together. Table 45 (Category A) shows that out of 212 hyperactive females, 30.7% are orgasmic through heterosexuality and 34.0% through masturbation, while non-orgasmic sex and no sexuality account only for 19.3% and 16% respectively. In the creative group (Table 45, Category B, N=267) observations and proportions similar to the hyperactive group can be observed. In Category C of the moderately active group (N=285), there is a tendency for the reverse: 9.8% for orgasmic, 2.5% for masturbation, 33.0% for non-orgasmic sex, and 54.7% for no sexuality. But the reverse trend is almost total in the inactive group (N-719, Category D of Table 45): practically no orgasm of any kind, some non-orgasmic sexuality (17.0%), and the bulk (82.0%) have completely given up sex. Table 45 therefore demonstrates that hyperactive/creative senior females are sexually active and orgasmic, and generally inactive senior females are sexually inactive.

Is the reverse also true, i.e., are most orgasmic women hyperactive-creative? This is demonstrated in Table 46. Out of 190 orgasmic women (Category 1), 34.2% are hyperactive, 48.5% are creative, 14.7% are moderately active, and only 2.6% are inactive. Orgasm through masturbation (Category 2) shows almost the same results as orgasm through heterosexuality (Category 1). The 281 heterosexual non-orgasmic women (Category 3) shows mixed results, although the trend was toward inactivity. Out of 836 non-sexual women (Category 4 of Table 46), the bulk (70.6%) are couch potatoes, and there is practically no hyperactive-creative among them (4.0% and 6.7%) although 18.7% show limited activity.

The conclusion from Tables 45 and 46 is that the great majority of hyperactive women and even more so of creative women are orgasmic, while the great majority of inactive women are non-sexual. And reversely the great majority of orgasmic women are hyperactive and even more so creative, while the great majority of non-sexual women are inactive. It is to be noted that women with non-orgasmic sexuality occupy an intermediate position, but with a definite tendency toward inactivity. To be noted also is that orgasm through masturbation gives women the same hyperactivity/creativity as heterosexual orgasm.

The close relationship between hyperactivity/creativity and orgasm on one side, between inactivity and non-sexuality on the other side is striking. This is true for senior men as well as senior women.

There are however differences between men and women. Proportionally speaking, there are more hyperactive-creative men than women: 59.5% of senior men are hyperactive-creative, and only 32.3% of women are. This is almost a proportion of two-to-one. This should not make us conclude that men are more hyperactive-creative than women. The truth is that senior men were already "on the job" as many of them kept doing what they were doing before senior age, or at least kept their job partially, while women were out of a job when their family responsibilities were terminated and had to look for a new job. It is much easier to stay on the same job than to look for a new career. This is well demonstrated in Table 47. Among the 971 men with various activities in senior age, almost two-thirds kept their old job (partially or totally) while only one-third looked for a new activity. Among the 764 women with various activities in senior age, we find the reverse. Only one-third kept their old job while almost two-thirds looked for a new activity. It is therefore understandable that only 268 out of 1239 senior males (21.6%) are inactive, while 719 out of 1483 senior women (48.8%) are inactive.

Historical Review of Sexuality in Senior Age

This relationship in old age between hyperactivity-creativity on one side and orgasm on the other (Tables 43-46) is puzzling to say the least and leaves one wondering about this relationship. Are seniors orgasmic because they are hyperactive-creative, or are they hyperactive-creative because they are orgasmic? To put it differently, is hyperactivity-creativity an aspect of orgasmic sexuality, or is orgasmic sexuality an aspect of hyperactivity-creativity? Which comes first is a difficult question to answer. A third possibility is that neither one comes first—both are a fused unity which is a total aspect of the individual personality, maybe genetic, maybe cultural, or maybe natural. Whatever the relationship, it is obvious that they go together. Sexuality and even more so, orgasmic sexuality, is the most intense pleasure to which a human being can be exposed to. This is especially true in senior citizens where sexuality is 'free' love because it has been liberated from all previous obligations such as fear of or desire for pregnancy, hormonal activity, lack of privacy, interference with other activities such as a job, etc. Sexuality becomes a 'free' pleasure in senior age, a pure pleasure that one indulges in when it is desired, or stays away from when not attracted to it. It cannot be denied, however, that orgasmic sexuality is much more than a pleasure in some senior citizens, notwithstanding the intensity of the pleasure. Far beyond pleasure, it is associated with an active and creative life, it is life itself in its most intense form. This observation, as far as I know, has never been demonstrated statistically in such a large series as was done in this investigation, although it is very casually mentioned in the literature in isolated cases.

One can look at history to confirm the above observation. In reviewing the tenure of American presidents, I cannot help comparing President Nixon to President Clinton. The presidency of the former was dull and the latter was dynamic. The Nixon presidency was ordinary, like the rest of his life, which was filled with failures. It is true that he terminated the Vietnam War but this was the work of his interior secretary, Henry Kissinger. Clinton's presidency, on the contrary, was associated with the greatest economical expansion in the history of the United States. Yet, the sexual life of President Nixon was puritanistic to the highest degree and the sexual life of President Clinton was exactly the opposite. It is not necessary to review the personal life and the achievements of the other American presidents to find similar examples of 'dull' presidents associated with a puritanistic life and 'dynamic' presidents associated with sexual liberties or even sexual scandals. Jack Kennedy is another example. Jackie Mason, the New York comedian, was well aware of the above, and humorously suggested that specific laws should be made with special provisions for sexual liberties to presidents in order to increase their performance during their tenure. I wonder how much of a joke is this suggestion!

Past history reveals similar observations. Prophet Mohammed is the founder of Islam. His fundamental religious concepts certainly have contributed in making Islam the largest religion in the world and the only religion that is still expanding. Yet, Mohammed's life is notorious for the number of his wives and mistresses. His concepts of sexuality, as mentioned in the Koran (Muslim Holy Book), must have played a definite role in making him and Islam a success. I wonder if there is there some teaching to the puritanistic Judeo-Christian concept of sexuality: prophet Mohammed stated that no woman in Islam should remain a virgin!

Among the people that were at the origin of Judaism, King Solomon is the founder of the Jewish state in antiquity. Having to deal with Jewish tribes that were deeply divided and surrounded by enemies that were much greater in number, one may wonder how King Solomon managed to create and maintain the State of Israel. Yet, the largest harem recorded in history is the one of King Solomon. His "Song of Songs," chanted every Friday night in Jewish temples, compares the relation between God and man to a sexual orgasm. One may wonder if his achievements as a monarch did not parallel his sexual achievements.

Julius Caesar is the military genius of antique Rome. His sexual life with Cleopatra and other women is well recorded in history.

Charlemagne consolidated European Christianity after the fall of the Roman Empire. Rome appreciated his religious achievements and easily closed its eyes to the number of his wives and mistresses.

The Turkish monarchs built an empire almost as great as the Roman Empire. Suleiman the Magnificent and his successors extended the limits of their empire and even threatened to destroy the Christian world. Yet, these monarchs were as famous for their harems as they were for their conquests.

Emperor Napoleon was the greatest military genius in history. As long as he had an active sexual life he was victorious in all his military campaigns. Then he married Princess Josephine from Austria whom he fell in love with. The Empress was not faithful to him, but he remained faithful to her and thus became sexually frustrated. I wonder about the parallel between his military successes and early sexual freedom on one side and his political/military failures and sexual frustrations later on in life on the other side. One is left to wonder how world history would have been modified if Napoleon had, in some way, resumed his early sexual activity, or if Empress Josephine had been in love with him and had remained faithful to him.

Catherine of Russia is definitely the founder of the Russian Empire. She was also the greatest art collector in the world. Yet, she remained sexually active and diversified to the end of her long life with the greatest number of lovers recorded in history. She even devised an elaborate and proficient system to keep steady the flow of her lovers.

Princess Diana from England is definitely the most famous contemporary figure in England and even outside of England. Yet, her liberated sexuality is slowly coming out into the open.

In order to understand puritanistic Christianity it would be desirable to look at it from an historical point of view. Early Christianity originated among Roman slaves and expanded as the Roman Empire started to fall. At that time, Roman citizens indulged in orgies with abundant sex and drinking. For instance, when a wealthy Roman, mostly a "nouveau riche," was hosting a party, beautiful courtesans in a side room were available to guests. The number of slaves was getting larger and larger, and the disparity of their way of life as compared to the Roman citizens was becoming abysmal. The freed slaves were no better off because there was no work for them and they were living on government subsidies, mostly free food. Sex was becoming so easily available, thanks to the imported female slaves, that even Roman ladies became sexually frustrated and started to solicit sex either from strangers or from male slaves. At that time, Christianity, which so far had a limited number of adepts, started to expand by preaching a heavenly life after death, and completely condemned wine and sex as sinful, as obstacles to a union with God, as degrading to the human soul, and as a sinful indulgence to flesh. It is fundamental to stress that the Christian church originally condemned sex in all its forms. The church barely recommended marriage, which led to sex, to bringing into the world children and exposing them to sinful activities.

Instead, early Christians recommended a purified sexless life on earth for the sole purpose of preparing ourselves to join God. It is only later on that it became obvious that it was better to keep bringing children into this world, otherwise Pagans would take over. But, the Christian rules were strict. Sex only for the purpose of procreation, and **no** other purpose. What was called carnal satisfaction or pleasure in sex by touch and for the purpose of reaching orgasm was considered a horrible sin and a betrayal of God. The Christian priesthood (male priests or nuns) never married and of course had no sex. These basic puritanistic rules have barely changed since. Of course, cheating and scandals (most of them unpublicized) were more and more frequent and included the highest Catholic hierarchy, even Popes (A Treasury of Royal Scandals, Michael Farquhar, Penguin Books, 1995). My point is that nobody has ever proven that these non-puritanistic religious figures were less of achievers than the puritanistic ones. After the split of Christianity into two parts, namely Catholicism and Protestantism, each side of the split returned to Puritanism, although non-Catholic priests were allowed to marry. Both remained puritan. The Roman legions of antique Rome represented a very disciplined and efficient army. And so was regulated the very liberal sexual behavior they took in the conquered lands.

The Western world, composed mostly of Christians, has a tendency to forget that Puritanism is purely Western. This sexually restrictive attitude of the Western world does not exist in the rest of the world. When the Spaniards landed in South America five centuries ago, they were surprised (and delighted!) to see how casual the natives were about sex. Sex with unmarried or even married women was not an insult to anybody's honor and not a sin, it was casual. These Spaniards who, when in Spain, had their sexual life dreadfully restricted by the Catholic church which used the

Inquisition when necessary, jumped all the way into this sexual freedom of South America and practically every South American native woman they could put their hands on was sired, so that the current South American population is largely the progeny of native women and Spaniards (Before Sexuality, D.M. Halperin et al. Princeton University Press, Princeton, N.J. 1990; Sex in History, R. Tannahill, Scarborough House/Publishers, 1992). The Spanish church was of course active all over South America, and attempted to convert all the Indians to Catholicism. But the Church closed its eyes to the sexual freedom of the Spaniards for the simple reason that sexual freedom in South America was well known all over Spain and was a stimulus for Spanish youth to join the Spanish army (Conquistadors) for the South American conquest. My impression is that this sexual freedom contributed to the conquest of the large continents of South and Central America by very few Spaniards. This was the greatest conquest in the history of mankind by so few soldiers and was associated with the greatest sexual freedom recorded in history.

The highest authoritative figure who has put Christian doctrine on a sound basis, Saint Augustine, did not have an exemplary sexual life until conversion and one may wonder if he would have been so productive had he abstained from sex before his revelation.

The Catholic priesthood is currently faced with sexual scandals. Not that these scandals are that great in number. With celibacy imposed on Catholic priests, a small percentage of such scandals is to be expected. The only difference is that now they have become publicized. This celibacy, which may have been justified during early Christianity, may presently be easing. I wonder if the current repression, imposed by the high Catholic hierarchy to the faulting priests, is the real answer. It may be better to revise the concept of celibacy and accept that one can have sex without renouncing God. The policy of maintaining celibacy, so that Catholic priests and nuns do not have heirs, and thus keeping and increasing the wealth of the church within the church, may need to be revised.

In the art world, the association of creativity and sexual freedom is well known. The Renaissance (literally 'Rebirth'), which started in Italy at the end of the 16th century, was a return to the arts and to all kinds of freedoms including sexual freedom. The sexual freedom during the Italian Renaissance had no limits. In Italian nobility at that time almost everyone had one or more than one mistress with numerous illegitimate children.

Among modern artists, Picasso and Wright are known as much for their artistic creations as for their diversified sexual life. The sexual lives of the most notorious Hollywood artists are well documented in the news media.

The last point I want to discuss is the problem of the boss having an affair with his secretary. Our puritanistic society requires that these affairs remain condemned and repressed. They also remain secretive unless there is a scandal such as a pregnancy, abortion, murder, or simple blackmail. These scandals delight the news media, especially when the media is short of news. I am not making any judgment, nor am I giving any opinion. However, during my current study, I have come across quite a few cases of retired bosses, who were very successful in their businesses, and who also had hidden affairs, mostly with their secretaries, during their years of successful activity. In fact I came to recognize this type of retired boss with previous sexual affairs almost immediately: men or women in their seventies, healthy looking, not obese, still active and/or creative, always going for their medical check-up but without excess, and practicing some sport; these people are almost always orgasmic within or outside of marriage even as seniors. Currently, the boss-secretary sexual affairs are frowned upon, leading to false or confirmed accusations and to sexual harassment. My impression is that emotions and Puritanism should be kept out of it, and should be completely dismissed if between consenting individuals. Surprisingly, since strict rules and regulations on reporting sexual harassment have been promulgated, the number of reported cases has markedly diminished and practically disappeared. I doubt very much that the number of boss-secretary affairs has diminished; I think these affairs still have the same stimulating effect on the bosses and on the secretaries.

Without establishing any cause-to-effect relationship between sexuality and hyperactivity-creativity, let us just conclude that, from the large series presented here, and from the previous historical review, sexuality certainly is not only highly pleasurable but a very important factor in human activity and creativity. This is true not only in any age, but also as demonstrated here (Tables 43-46), in senior age.

Summary of all Previous Data on Senior Sexuality

Quite a few conclusions can be drawn from Tables 30-47 that tabulate sexual activity and inactivity in senior males and females. These conclusions are summarized as follows.

From a sexual point of view there are far less available senior men than senior women. Only one man in five is sexually inactive, while more than half the women are sexually inactive, both for lack of a sexual partner. A little more than half the women are therefore deprived of a sexual partner and this deprivation is spread more or less evenly among the different age population in women (Table 35).

Senior women are more individualized and selective in looking for sexual relationships than men (Tables 30-33). They are hesitant in approaching and in being approached although modern senior women are more forward than the previous generation. Women rarely have more than one sexual affair at a time or pay a man for sex, while men generously have affairs, easily turn to prostitutes, and occasionally indulge in more than one sex partner at a time.

In the senior community some men like to show off and exhibit sexuality beyond their real performance, while less women exhibit more sexual interest than they really have. Similar numbers of subjects want to look younger than their age.

From a sexual point of view it is apparent that not all seniors perform well. Out of 1236 men, 16.9% (Table 17) perform poorly (incomplete erection, incomplete or no ejaculation) leading to some frustration, and 19% of women are non-orgasmic in their heterosexuality. There is less frustration in women than in men side when there is non-orgasmic performance. However, while some senior men would like to perform more, only a few women do.

Sexual activity for purposes other than sexual desire is significant in the senior community. Among 1239 men, only a small fraction have sex to satisfy and/or keep a partner as a companion, while many more women have sex for the same purpose. In addition, many women declare that they are financially supported by their sexual partner, and would leave him if it were not for the support. There were very few men in that category.

Tables 17, 19 and 21give us the percentage of orgasm when masturbating. It is infrequent in men (4.6%), about the same prior to senior age and remains about the same all through senior age. The picture is completely different in women. Although orgasm through masturbation is also minimal in adulthood (4.7%), it increases significantly in senior age (average 11.9%). The percentage is erratic among different female age groups but is consistent with increased age (7.1% in the 55-59 age group; 13.7% in the 85+ age group).

Tables 19, 20, 21 show that there is an increased (and failed) attempt among senior men to perform more sexually. Among 1239 men, there were 117 cases of poor sexuality before age 55, with this number increasing to 210 after age 55 (an increase by 80%, Table 21). Table 19 also shows that there is a peak in the 70s. For women, the picture is completely different. Among 1483 women, 812 were non-orgasmic before age 55, with the number dropping to 281 after age 55, a two-third drop. The majority of women who were non-orgasmic before age 55 refused to continue non-orgasmic sex after age 55; the remaining third continued to be non-orgasmic in an uneven distribution among the different senior ages.

That sexual inactivity increases slowly in men and drastically in women, is obvious in Tables 19 and 21. Among 1239 men, 139 were sexually inactive before age 55; 257 (an increase of 65.9%) were inactive after age 55. Among 1483 women, 359 were sexually inactive before age 55; 836 (an increase of 125%) were inactive after age 55.

What can we conclude from the above observations?

1. Men who had been orgasmic before age 55, had a tendency to remain orgasmic. The persistence of orgasm is even more obvious among women. Therefore, orgasmic sexuality has a tendency to persist regardless of age, and this is specifically true for women.
2. Masturbation is very rare among adult and senior men, and is also in adult women; however the number of women who masturbate increases with age.
3. Although there is some decrease in sexual orgasms in men, women tended to give up sex altogether if it was not associated with climax.

The previous pages may give the impression that romance is gone from senior sexuality. Nothing is further from the truth. Their romance is just different from romance of the young, which is based on a frequent and prolonged type of sexuality, on the male courting the woman for sexual favors, and on a well-established protocol that can vary from one social class or culture to another, but has the strength of having been well established over many generations.

Senior romance can still respect this established protocol or can establish new ones. Men and women can be different from one another. Gentleness and gallantry, still active in old age, has a different tone. Gone is the 'macho' man. The reserve and shyness of women and the aggressive, forwardness of men no longer play an important role. Some men may still want to act the role of the young and adult but it does not always work. New roles are being explored that are more suitable to individual senior cases. Both men and women look essentially for companionship, some look for glamour in a relationship, and still others prefer the enjoyment of total or partial solitude. Although there is still some biological sex drive in men and in quite a few women who are still orgasmic, in general, the sexual drive is less intense then it was in younger years. Seniors can still enjoy each other's company, be together all day long, and even sleep together, and yet have a diminished and even a non-sexual life.

Many seniors keep or at least attempt to keep the old sexual approach. Even if they partially or totally fail, they try to keep the external appearance of young success and in this matter lie to themselves as well as others. These are the ones who are the main source of gossip about senior sexuality.

How to Analyze Senior Sexuality

We have shown that there is some relation between deteriorating health and sexual activity. The relation is not absolute, far from it, as we saw all kinds of different sexual activities in all kinds of different stages of health and age. In this chapter we will show that sexual hormones have markedly diminished or have even disappeared with advancing age, demonstrating therefore that sexual activity in seniors is not related to the presence or absence of sexual hormones.

We are left therefore in a quandary, wondering about the cause and reason, if any, of sexual activity in seniors. We will devise a new approach in order to understand this problem. In this and subsequent chapters we will attempt to analyze the causes of these differences: "Felix qui potuit causa rerum cognoscere = happy is the one who recognizes the cause of things."

We will study first all the factors that determine sexual activity in general, then we will center on the reasons for senior sexuality. Namely, we will study the following aspects of sexuality:

* Sexuality in animals and all the biological factors that determine it.
* Sexuality in prehistoric humans and how it differs from animal sexuality.
* Transition from animal to human sexuality. Why, how, and when it occurred.
*Differences between human male and female sexuality.
* Sexuality in senior men and women, and how different it is from adult or young.

It is essential to understand that nature has provided all living creatures with a mode of reproduction. Specifically, it provided all animals with reproductive organs. Only in the human species have these reproductive organs become sexual organs, or organs of sexual pleasure, and I would add more sexual organs than reproductive organs. Seniors are "stuck" with organs that are no longer reproductive but only sexual. The future of senior sexuality can be determined only in the light of past and present history of sexuality. It is only by determining what causes sexuality in other living groups (animals, prehumans, adult men and women), that we can ask what causes sexuality in seniors. Should seniors be motivated toward sexuality for the same or different reasons as other living groups? This problem is important because it is new in human history. Senior citizenry has appeared only recently in a large scale and is expanding at an increasing speed and the problems associated with such an expanding population, including their sexuality, need to be addressed.

Indeed, nature or evolution has provided us with reproductive organs for the sole purpose of reproduction. Olfactory hormones (pheromones) play an essential role in animal coital attraction, which is purely biological. In humans, the biological (hormonal) attraction has practically disappeared. Visual and tactile attractions which make the sexual attraction highly pleasurable has become of primary importance, far beyond reproductive sex. Sex has also become a union between two people. There is some kind of conflict between these two different goals. In seniors, reproduction and all the biology that goes with it has completely disappeared and left only are sexual pleasure and union between individuals. All male privileges of animal ancestry and partly maintained in Homo sapiens during his adulthood are to be reconsidered in senior age.

Description of the Male and Female Orgasm

The human male orgasm is easy to characterize: it is the climax following multiple sexual stimulations of the erect penis while penetrating the vaginal cavity. The rubbing of the erect penis against the vaginal mucosa is very stimulating while sperm accumulates in the seminal vesicles, prostatic canals and upper urethra. The sudden ejection of the sperm through the urethral canal produces an intense feeling or orgasm. This mode of ejaculation is physiological and has been present in the animal world for billions of years. The male orgasm can be considered biological and natural because it is a physiological phenomenon, leading to ejaculation that is necessary for reproduction. Reproduction is the ultimate and natural goal of male orgasm.

This ejaculatory process is practically identical in all mammals. It is unknown how much orgasm or sexual pleasure accompanies ejaculation in animals. What is certain is that the tonic and clonic spasms associated with human orgasm are never seen in animals, therefore giving the impression that there is ejaculatory relief rather than ejaculatory orgasm. One can conclude therefore that orgasm superimposed and associated with ejaculation is specific to the human species, and does occur without ejaculation. Inability to ejaculate means no orgasm.

Male and female orgasms are so different from each other that they barely deserve the same name (Table 49). The human female orgasm is a completely different matter. It is only by analogy that it is also called orgasm. Female orgasm is also called climax. The female orgasm does not fulfill any physiological function as it is not necessary for reproduction, as is male orgasm. Orgasmic, as well as non-orgasmic women, get pregnant the same way as long as the sperm is deposited into the upper vaginal cavity at a specific moment of the menstrual cycle.

In fact, continuous observations and research in the animal world have led many researchers to the conclusion that orgasm as observed in the human female does not exist at all in the animal world (Table 48). All one sees in non-human females is relief from male weight and male aggression immediately after ejaculation. Human female climax is not natural, whatever the word 'natural' means. It is a human acquisition, acquired late in human evolution. I would say it is characteristic of Homo (or rather Femina sapiens), like other human characteristics, such as language. Some women are more predisposed to it, others never heard of it. It is now time to describe and define female orgasm because many women do not know what it is.

Real female orgasm needs careful and gentle preparation by an experienced, loving and loved partner. It also needs a highly receptive female partner who knows how to communicate her desires. It is characterized by a spasm of the muscles surrounding the vaginal cavity and, in fact, all the muscles of the body, followed by general relaxation and a feeling of ecstasy. There may be a couple of vaginal spasms or as many as fifteen and even more. The state of ecstasy that follows is so impressive that a woman never forgets it. Her face and whole personality become 'illuminated.' The vaginal mucosa becomes more humid during the build-up and culminates in climax but there is no ejaculation of any kind as there is in men. I repeat that the human female is the only one in the animal world to have sexual climax.

Modern women are very open about producing sexual orgasm in themselves either through masturbation with their own fingers or using various instruments such as a vibrator. Lesbians can also stimulate each other by using various techniques.

The female climax is not a biological phenomenon and the emission of the egg by the human female does not require any orgasm and, in fact, does not even require a sexual act at all since the egg is spontaneously emitted on the 14th day of the menstrual cycle.

We can summarize the above as follows. Somehow during human evolution, and taking advantage of his anatomy and physiology as described above, the male of the human species automatically combined orgasm with ejaculation. While the female of the human species, because of her anatomy and physiology did not necessarily associate climax with each sexual act. Orgasm and climax are not animal in origin. They have been progressively built up during human evolution. The evolution of female climax is not complete yet. In general it can be stated that during the sexual act, the male automatically and easily reaches orgasm, while it is far from being so with the human female. These consequences are fundamental in male-female relationships and they determine the drama and the apotheosis of human culture in general.

Each gender finds advantages and disadvantages in these differences. The male, easily stimulated, quickly reaches ejaculation-orgasm, but since ejaculation is necessary for orgasm, he has to build up his sperm reserve for the next orgasm. Therefore, the average adult male has sex only once a day at most.

The contention of multiple orgasms in humans is mentioned only in the lay sexual literature without much scientific authenticity. Some males have the ability to interrupt the sexual act in the middle of ejaculation, reserving the rest of the ejaculate for the next sexual act during which they complete the ejaculation. What they really had are two (rarely three) incomplete and unsatisfactory orgasms during the same sexual setting, instead of a complete and satisfactory one. Some males like to brag about such a performance and the lay sexual literature has capitalized on it. What really happens is that the human male often has difficulty delaying his ejaculation orgasm either because he wants to extend the number of pleasurable thrusts, or, as we will see later, because he is waiting for his female partner to reach her own climax. One thing is sure, the human male can hardly fake an orgasm because he has to produce the proof of it (the ejaculated sperm).

Sexual climax in the human female is not associated with any biological function. It is elusive, takes time to build up and is hard to reach. Sexual pornography describes women actively involved in all kinds of sexual postures in order to reach a climax. In reality the conditions surrounding the female climax require skill, patience and intimacy with a specific sexual partner. The female climax requires a close cooperation with the male partner who makes it his duty and obligation to guide the female partner in reaching her climax. Putting aside all the advertising and fictitious stories about female climax, I learned a few basic facts during my career as a marriage counselor. I do not know any woman who reached a climax during her first coitus especially if it was with a stranger she barely knew, even if she previously reached orgasm through masturbation. Most women express indifference, pain, and/or embarrassment regarding their first experience. It takes a long time and a skilled partner to progressively overcome the fear of sexuality and progressively build up the necessary atmosphere for a climax. Many women go through life, married or not, without ever reaching orgasm, and many others have barely experienced it. Quite a few researchers when studying female climax are satisfied by simply asking the female subject whether or not she reached climax and how often. Embarrassingly, the women most often says yes.

I always did more and always asked the subject to describe in detail the nature of her climax. This is how I learned that a large number of women, maybe half of them, confuse climax with something else. Some women are thrilled by the intimacy with the male even without orgasm and they think that is all there is. Some women confuse the male orgasm as their own climax. Some others are so concerned about producing an orgasm in the male partner that they consider this a great accomplishment and are satisfied with it. Some women are sincerely in love with their male partner and, as unbelievable as it seems, are highly content with him being attracted to them and being sexually happy. Finally some learn to fake a climax because they know that it builds up the ego of their partner or they simply become bored and tired and even physically irritated by the successive thrusts and want to put an end to it. It is much easier for a woman to fake orgasm than it is for a man. By the way, women faking orgasm rarely works, at least not for long. My opinion about multiple orgasms in women is the same as multiple orgasms in men; they are false, incomplete, or faked orgasms, and mostly good for cheap publicity or pornography literature.

Transition to Senior Sexuality

Coitus is the sexual union of two genitalia of opposite sex. In humans, the sexual act, especially for those who meet for the first time, is preceded by noncoital sexuality usually called presex, petting, necking, and other nicknames. It usually involves one partner touching any part of the partner's body with lips or hands. This presex can be elaborate especially in teenagers and sometimes it comprises the whole act, as it may or may not lead to male or female orgasm.

In seniors presex, or whatever one wants to call it, is markedly reduced in technique and in time. The reason is that usually the female has already consented to the sexual act. Therefore the male partner does not have to convince or seduce or overcome any resistance. The woman often takes the initiative and when the male consents, he is directly invited to her bed. Rarely do women request an elaborate preparation to which they may or may not participate. Rarely would a woman be satisfied with necking, as teenagers would do. 'Cock teasing' is not on the senior woman's agenda. Because the woman is as much interested in a relationship as she is in sex, she is often satisfied in leading her partner to sex and orgasm even if she does not necessarily look for climax herself.

The human male and female cycles do not necessarily coordinate timewise or go together. One may terminate before the other. Most of the time it is the man who finishes first (remnant of animal ancestry where ejaculation quickly follows penetration) and the woman has not even started her erotic cycle. The male ejaculates and stops his thrusts before the woman gets her climax and vaginal spasms. Frequently human sex goes the wrong way: for the male, quick penetration, ejaculation, and withdrawal, while the female has barely started, if at all, or the woman is close to climax but left cold and twisting in the air after the male partner ejaculates and withdraws. The coordination or lack of coordination between the male and female cycle is the ecstasy or the tragedy of human sex. It is the art or the lack of it in human sexuality.

On the other extreme one can have a patient, skillful, loving coordination of a progressive arousal between the two partners, terminating in a simultaneous orgasm with the two parties embracing long after their climax. Fool is the human individual who thinks that such ecstasy is natural. It is not. Fool is the individual who thinks that if the ecstasy is not reached, it is his/her fault: it is both their faults. Neither of the partners should expect the other to be ready for it. It is only in sex videos that this comes spontaneously. For a couple to both reach climax, patience, mutual confidence, training and practice and most of all love are needed. In my long career as a marriage and sex counselor, what I heard most often were complaints from each one about the other.

Between these two extremes are all kinds of intermediary stages in human sexuality. There is the frigid woman who never had an orgasm in her life, who develops a perfect indifference to it, and considers sex a duty. The greatest loss in a woman's life is to be indifferent to sex or, worse, repulsed by her sexual partner. It will affect all her life, including senior life.

Then, there is the man who eliminates all preparation, has as few thrusts as possible for a quick ejaculation, turns his back, goes to sleep, or goes away (slam, 'bam, thank you Ma'am). This man is labeled a playboy and/or promiscuous, and measures his sexual success by the highest number of sexual partners he may have.

None of these behaviors are related to the level of sex hormones; this sexual diversity is purely cerebral. I went through this long list to find out how these various attitudes are modified when citizens reach old age without hormones or any biological drive. No more desire for pregnancy, or practicing birth control in order to avoid it. No more children around to interfere with any sexual activity, no more coming home from work tired and unable to have sex before going to sleep, no more getting up early in the morning and leaving without having sex. Weekends are no longer for recovering from the fatigue acquired during the week but for hobbies. The unstable equilibrium that determined sex in adulthood has completely collapsed, and all the previous excuses have to be replaced with reality. If the couple were working and now both are retired, there is plenty of time for sex and everything else. The real male and female personality now appear naked. This new reality results in many different outcomes. For loving couples who step into seniorhood the transition is very smooth and they keep living the way they lived previously, sexually or otherwise; they may have more or less sex than before, it does not matter. Their intimacy has not been disturbed and it may even be reinforced because they have more time for each other.

There are couples for whom the job, children, and fear of pregnancy, only hide their lack of love. Seniorhood brings their deep personality to the open. The couple may start to argue, or they may live apart like strangers in the same house, separate rooms, separate everything.

It is in the field of senior sexuality that challenges can be more radical. Some may lose interest in sex, others may have increased interest, for others it remains the same. Some that never made advances now feel free to make them. Some would like to maintain the usual sexual position, others to explore new ones. Often it is the man, and not the woman, who likes to keep things as usual. Many women lose interest in sex after menopause but just as many like to innovate because of the new freedom from menstruation, from birth control, from having children around, etc. All these factors inhibited women more than men.

The Appearance of Beauty as a Human Mode of Sexual Attraction

What makes two creatures of the opposite sex attract each other from a sexual point of view, and create in them a desire for coitus? Is one sex (male or female) more attracted sexually to the other?

Because the human mode of sexual stimulation (visual, tactile, mental and emotional) exists in both sexes, their sexual attraction is reciprocal. In animals there is no reciprocity. That the animal female sexually attracts the male but not vice-versa, and that humans of both genders can sexually attract each other, is the crucial difference between animals and humans. It should be clearly specified however that although it works both ways, i.e., both human male and female stimulate each other, it is more the female that stimulates the male by sight and touch, than the reverse. At any rate the remnants of this difference in human species are important in understanding human sexuality (Table 48, 49). Whatever part of the female body is exposed or hidden becomes sexually attractive. This is how the concept of beauty was born in humans and how animal/human differences appear. Beauty is essentially the physical attraction of the female body, concentrated mostly on facial features. Physical beauty does not exist in animals. In the animal mounting position all female backs look alike and all that concerns the female is the weight of the male on her back.

During early human evolution the olfactory attraction of the animal female was progressively replaced by the visual attraction of the human female face. This transition took two million years to occur (from "Lucy" of two million years ago to the Neanderthal) and was facilitated by the transition of the animal sexual posture to the human sexual posture. In summary, female 'beauty' has become the sexual attraction in humans, completely replacing the animal pheromones.

Oh, how I do miss the beautiful complexion I had when I was young. My mother taught me about make-up and I mastered the art quickly. I worked in the dress department of a famous store and I always was well dressed without spending much money. I always knew how to expose or hide parts of my anatomy, my breasts, my legs, my thighs. When I was wearing a short skirt, all I had to do was sit down and I could follow the eyes of the boys trying to see how high they could look under my skirt. But it was in my bikini bathing suit that I attracted the eyes of all the guys. Now, half a century later, it is all gone. I tried plastic surgery, but it did not improve my appearance. It was a waste of money. I have become allergic to make-up products, and beauticians have almost completely destroyed my hair with all kinds of chemicals. I do not go to the beautician anymore. My hair is now OK but it is all white. I do not feel the need to expose my legs anymore. I got married a few times and I had many sexual affairs, but it is over now. My last affair was two years ago with a 78 year old man, but he could not do much sexually speaking. I guess my beautiful life, sexual and otherwise, is over now. What a pity. It was good as long as it lasted. For a woman to be young and beautiful is real life.

Q: Have you tried any sexual stimulants?

A: No. I heard that Viagra works only for men. I am now investigating the growth hormone. I heard it does miracles.

The fundamental characteristic of female beauty is that it is transitory, and starts to fade near female menopause as the female ages and wrinkles start to spread over her face and body. Sexual attraction based solely on physical beauty diminishes, although there are numerous exceptions as will be discussed later. Up to a century ago aging had never been a problem for females (as well as males) because the population barely survived beyond their forties. Most women died without many wrinkles on their face and could be considered sexually attractive up to the end of their life, so mankind safely connected sexual attraction and physical (mostly facial) beauty.

Then senior age appeared with the average life span jumping from 48 to 79 years of age for women and from 46 to 74 in men. This is a two-third increase in their life span, with a promise to get higher. Now the premenopausal life of a woman (from 12 to 50) is almost equal to her postmenopausal life (from 50 to 79) and will even be higher in the future.

If there is going to be sexual attraction in postmenopausal women and certainly there will be at least for many of them, sexual attraction will not necessarily be based on physical beauty.

Physical beauty is not the only mode of attraction that can be used by the human female (Femina sapiens) in order to attract the human male (Homo sapiens). In the prehuman period lasting two million years, as posture became fully erect, early humans looked at their genital organs which were now fully exposed and finally realized that there were important differences. The male had two testicles and a penis which, at the slightest touch, increased in size and became erect. The female had–nothing. Since early time and up to the present time women have been suffering of 'penis envy' (Sigmund Freud). Therefore, they made a mystery of hiding 'nothing' behind a fig leaf or whatever clothing they wore. This picture has barely changed. What women were hiding behind a fig leaf or clothing became a mystery and from the beginning men have wondered what women hide behind their clothes. "Ontogeny is a short phylogeny" said Stephen J. Gould. Early in life young girls are told to hide their genitals as they grow up, with the concept of hiding a valuable treasure. After puberty, especially as their breasts blossom and their whole body becomes beautiful, each pubescent girl imagines that there is another inaccessible 'inner sanctum' that every man is looking after.

Now we have the complete picture of an adolescent girl as she approaches adulthood. A sense of physical beauty, mostly facial beauty and the feeling of a hidden treasure, the access to which is to be limited, delayed, made difficult to approach because very valuable.

This concept of physical beauty and inner treasure starts to wear off during adulthood and is practically gone in most women when they become seniors. For many, not only is the physical beauty gone, but the concept of inner treasure is gone too. Some women may keep believing in the inner treasure but as less and less men look for it, it is no longer a mystery.

The 'magic' of being sexually penetrated, of a highly valuable treasure sought after by every man, is practically all gone. The senior woman no longer resists sex, but approaches it more casually; she no longer considers it a highly valuable favor. In fact she may even be very glad that a man is looking after her, from a sexual point of view. This is the reason why the role between the two opposite sex is frequently reversed in senior age. The woman has 'nothing' to hide and to be sought after, and now it is the man who holds a valuable treasure. The sexual approach to a woman is much simpler and, if so inclined, she will make the approach easier and even make the first approach. Of course, if not interested, the woman will cut off any approach from the start. The increasing number of women and the diminishing number of men accelerate this radical change.

As a gynecologist I remember the tremendous resistance of teenagers and early adult women to any gynecological examination, and the relative casualty of it in senior age. Except for spinsters, vaginal examination in a senior is no different from examination of any other part of their body.

The Reversal of Roles in Senior Sexuality

I have been happily married all my life. I am now 77 years old. Then my wife passed away three years ago. She died of generalized cancer. A few weeks before she passed away, when it became known that she was terminal, I started becoming the target of some bizarre attention. I could have done without it, considering how preoccupied and occupied I was with my dying wife. Senior ladies, either divorced, widows, or single, started to call me on the phone, or approached me directly and, I will not hesitate to say, harassed me. These ladies were either vague acquaintances or completely unknown to me. They proposed to help me anyway they could. Most of them, I found out, were just fishing for a companion. Some were trying to be vaguely polite and compassionate but others were aggressive and direct about being available and willing to move in with me. Immediately after the funeral, it got worse. Some, completely unknown to me and to my family paid us a "courtesy" visit during the mourning period. Now I barely answer these calls.

After one year as a widower, I tried to move to some kind of senior community. I visited a popular one and the manager took me around for a tour. Obviously it must have been written on my face that I was "available", or the manager must have spread the rumor of a male availability. I sincerely declare that I was frightened by the looks ladies of all ages were giving me.

Fortunately, I have close friends who respect my year of mourning and who are genuinely concerned about me and delicately and gently try to match me with some lady I may be compatible with. But it will take a long time.

This is the beginning of the third year I am alone. Rather than looking for a companion I have developed important hobbies. I play bridge two to three times a week, I do a lot of reading and I am very interested in history. I travel a lot. I feel that I will soon be ready for a female companion but I am happy to find that there is choice, maybe even too much choice. I am not in a rush and I finally started to go out with a lady a few years younger than I am. We both are trying to determine how compatible we can be, how we can match our interests, our schedules, and most of all how to respect each other's privacy. We are now sexually involved but we quickly found out that there are many problems in our mutual relationship that need to be addressed. It will take time. One thing is certain: although I sometimes miss my wife terribly and occasionally I feel lonely, most of the time I appreciate my freedom of movement. It is a tremendous feeling to do whatever I feel like doing, and go wherever I want to without accounting to anybody. I am not ready to compromise or give up this new freedom.

This reversal of roles between senior men and women can sometimes reach comical proportions with women in the hunt for a male partner and men embarrassed by their sometimes aggressive approach, and trying to avoid and hide from them. Samantha (see Introduction) is wrong and an old man can become attractive from the sexual point of view. As incredible as it may seem the period of a man's life when he is the most looked after by women is in senior age. It is too bad that in senior age the sexual capability of men is often diminished. As the French say: "Si jeunesse savait, si viellesse pouvait : if the young knew, if the old could." As we saw previously, modern sexual stimulants will take care of increasing male impotence.

Is There Beauty in Old Age?

It is only after having described sexual attraction in animals, prehumans, and adult humans that we can finally approach the prospect of sexual attraction in seniors. To look beautiful is to look young and the younger you look, the more beautiful you are: no woman beyond her twenties wins a beauty pageant, and all the pictures of women in magazines are of very young looking women. Since aging women never existed previously to such an extent, the concept of beauty excluded very few women.

According to the classic concept, an aging woman will still be beautiful only in the measure that she looks younger than she is. The art of cosmetics, clothing, and plastic surgery is the art of looking young. Today the average life span of a woman is 79 to 80 years and, if senior women want to look beautiful, they have to try harder to look young. Another approach would be to redefine beauty, as far as senior women are concerned, in a definition not necessarily connected with the beauty of youth. Does a senior woman have to look young in order to be beautiful? That is the question!

Sam is 81 years old. For a man of this age, he looks very good. He is tall, slim, walks straight and he plays tennis every day of the week, including weekends. His only concern used to be complete baldness, but he corrected it through a hair transplant at his wife's suggestion. He does a lot of facial massage and when you look at him he looks fifty, at most sixty.

His only problem is his wife. Although she is eight years younger, she looks at least ten years older. She had a nose job, then a face lift, but nothing worked. The tragedy is that she has become so obsessed with the wrinkles all over her face and body, that she lives in her house in complete darkness. There is a little light coming from the outside through heavy curtains and at night there is only a dim light in her house. She imagines that this way nobody will see her and she will not see her wrinkles. She barely goes out, and only at night to restaurants that she knows have dim lighting.

Her husband keeps reassuring her that he loves her as she is, and that the only reason he had a hair transplant was because she insisted on it. He ends up being the only one to go outside for shopping or any other activity. They both have a regular sexual life, frequently orgasmic, about once a week. But she insists that it should be in complete darkness. The only solution that Sam sees is that he should age further in his own appearance.

Let us say right here that men are not as obsessed with youth and beauty as women are. Mostly they passively go along with this concept, although the 'macho' man feels more virile with a young and beautiful woman than an old one. Since the woman has to be sexually attractive mostly in her youth, which is the time to secure a permanent sexual partner, emphasis is on youth and beauty, and it becomes almost second nature for women to keep looking young and beautiful for the rest of their adult life. Then, senior age appeared on a wide scale, leaving these senior citizens in a quandary as to what is now sexual attraction for them, as they are no longer young and beautiful in a young way. Should they fight for youth and beauty through hair styling, pedicures, manicures, jewelry, clothing, plastic surgery, or should they give up the fight for youth and beauty, and for the sexual attraction that goes with it? Finally, should they look for a mode of sexual attraction that is specific to their own age, discarding youth and beauty or rather discarding the current concepts of beauty associated with youth? Should a senior woman stop hiding wrinkles on her face to keep looking young and classically beautiful, or should she be comfortable with them and even proud of them? In support of this last point, it is important to stress that these concepts of youth and beauty are subjective rules, that have been found to be expedient by the young female generation for the purpose of attracting male attention. Young women know too well, and if they do not know they will learn later on the hard way, that to be young and beautiful does not make a relationship, any kind of relationship, permanent. Unless the male-female relationship is maintained at a superficial level whereby only the looks and the appearance constitute the relationship, the relationship falls apart. A deep and long lasting relationship calls on more profound values that goes far beyond any physical attraction on the part of the female as well as the male.

Among senior couples living together, some were married before or after retirement, and some just lived together. These people, although in love, do not consider sex a necessary component of their relationship, regardless of whether they are sexually active or not. Among the group with intimate relationship and no sex, half have been sleeping together for years and would not think of using separate beds.

The impression one gets from this review is that in senior age, the concept of love, intimacy, orgasmic and non-orgasmic sex, beauty as such, and beauty associated with youth are to be thoroughly reconsidered, for some seniors at least. These concepts have been created by and for the young and adult. Seniors are free to inherit or adopt them, or make any combination of them, but seniors are also free to reject these concepts totally or partially. The majority of the young and adults think that to be young and beautiful the young way is to be sexually attractive. They are free to think so because it applies to their age and complexion. But they are absolutely wrong to think that absence of youth and absence of a beautiful complexion makes a senior sexually unattractive and sexually excluded. Unless, of course, seniors think the same way. In fact, those seniors who think the same way, confirm the young and adults in their personal way of thinking. Nothing is more irritating to a young woman than a senior woman comfortable with her physical appearance.

Although many young and adult men and women think they are sexually more attractive to senior men and women than a senior man or woman would be; although many young and adult imagine that their youthful appearance is a strong asset when relating to seniors, our next study and statistics demonstrate that it is not so. The only exception is when a senior looks for a prostitute, it is true that she is much younger. Even so, I wonder what would happen if senior prostitutes were as easily available to senior men as the younger ones. When looking for a permanent companion, seniors rarely look for a younger age and rather look for senior partners.

Senior Men Attraction to Younger Women

A woman finds herself sexually attractive in the measure that she appears beautiful but this is not always true for men. The male face and body appear to age more slowly than females possibly because the male climacteric appears later and is less pronounced than female menopause. Men quickly learn that their wrinkles count much less in their life than they count in senior women's life. The reason is that sexual attraction of a man is based on such sexual performance as erection and its maintenance, and ejaculation more than on physical appearance. Besides, spiritual and emotional values come into play, diminishing the value of physical beauty which count much less in seniorhood than in adulthood and in youth.

The meaning and the value of physical beauty is therefore more important to women themselves than it is to men. It is not a male imperative as it is a female imperative. Not many women realize that, regardless of age, their appearance is more important to them as women than it is to men. Men give much less importance to female beauty than women think they do. If women were aware that their physical appearance was not that important to men, they certainly would spend less time and money on it. In fact women do not realize, especially married women, that the continuous concern about their physical appearance is, if anything, exasperating to men. Of course, the opposite, i.e., neglected appearance can also be damaging. It is true that physical appearance can be important at first, but afterwards it loses its value, and the value of a nice personality becomes predominant. This becomes much more important in senior age. The senior woman who approaches a senior man with a tremendous concern for her physical appearance, who hides her wrinkles behind excessive make up, who wears flashy clothing with a short skirt, who is seductive and aggressive in her approach or, on the contrary, plays very hard to get, will barely make it to first base and, if she does, she never goes beyond. It is unfortunate that not too many senior women realize this and hold onto the concept inherited from an earlier age where physical attraction and seduction are the keys to success.

The belief that old men are sexually attracted only by young and pretty women is widespread, although it is a rare event published mostly by the news media when a rich old man marries his maid and leaves all his money to her after he dies. Any young woman who dreams of such luck, better buy some lottery tickets because she has more chance of winning the jackpot than meeting such a man. Practically all wealthy old men who remarry a very young spouse always protect their wealth either with a careful will or a detailed prenuptial agreement. A wealthy senior woman who marries a young man "out of sudden love" is even rarer. In our series of 3396 cases we did not encounter a case of wealthy senior men or women marrying very young men or women.

Figure 8 shows how sixty-three available senior men and sixty-six available senior women have selected a new partner (remarriage or new companionship) in terms of difference in age. Figure 8A shows that most men selected a spouse or companion from five years older to ten years younger than them; twelve selected a new spouse or companion more than ten years younger, and four selected a new spouse or companion that is much older. Figure 8B shows how an available senior woman selects a new partner (remarriage or new companionship) in terms of difference in age. Most senior women had a new spouse or companion from five years younger to fifteen years older than them; six had a companion or spouse more than fifteen years older, and one more than twenty years younger.

Figure 9 is very interesting. It shows age differences of couples with a longstanding marriage or relationship that had been established well before they stepped into seniorhood. Figure 9A shows that the majority of men select a spouse from five years older to fifteen years younger than them long before becoming seniors. A few selected a spouse older than them, and a few selected a spouse more than twenty years younger. Similarly Figure 9B shows that the majority of women selected a spouse from five years younger to fifteen years older than them long before becoming seniors. There were only a couple of cases outside these ranges.

By comparing Figures 8 and 9 one can conclude that seniors are no different from the younger generation in terms of difference in age with a new partner. One observes in seniors the same differences in age between partners as one observes in younger age. The concept that seniors, especially senior men, look for younger partners because they are sexually more attractive, is completely erroneous. Sexual attraction is not the only factor that enters the mind of the senior (or the younger for that matter) when looking for a permanent partner.

There are some differences however between Figures 8 and 9, i.e., between adults and seniors when selecting a partner. Figure 8 shows that when a senior male selects a new partner, he is on average 4.5 years older; and when a senior woman selects a new partner, she is on average 4.6 years younger. Figure 9 shows that when the partnership is established well before senior age, the man is 6.0 years older and the woman 5.3 years younger, on average. Therefore, in opposition to younger age, seniors are narrowing the gap and appear to prefer a partner closer to their age. A very elevated difference in age can be seen in isolated seniors that are not seen in adults. This is understandable because seniors, being older, have more choice in selecting younger partners and can get involved in rare situations of an old senior with a very young bride. We had three such cases in our population: two senior men and one senior lady marrying or getting involved with a partner more than thirty years younger.

In Figures 8 and 9 we reported only stable relationships, either remarriage or stable companionship. We have not included the cases where seniors get involved in casual affairs like senior men who visit female prostitutes or more rarely senior women getting involved with male prostitutes.

Figure 10 studies the difference in age between **sexual** partners in senior age. This figure is different from Figure 8, which does not necessarily show sexual activity. Figures 10A and 10B do not show much difference from Figures 9A and 9B, and are representative of sexual activity in senior life. The conclusion, therefore, is that, when selecting a sexual partner, the senior citizen does not look for a younger partner than at any previous age. The concept that a senior citizen looks for a sexual partner that is much younger is not true, and they do not necessarily consider that a much younger partner will make sex more stimulating, or easier, or of any different quality. In fact, the opposite is true, at least in the three cases reported here, of extreme differences in age. The mismatching in these three cases is pitiful, and their sexual life is a disaster. The three of them hesitantly acknowledged that they could not keep up with the sexual demands of the partner and two of them (one senior man and the senior lady) were aware that the younger spouses were having outside affairs.

I am now 66 years old. I have been divorced for 20 years. Last year, I had a triple coronary bypass. I never had a real heart attack but I was suffering from constant chest pain and x-ray studies on my heart showed complete blockage of my coronary arteries. The surgical operation did not go too well and I had a second operation. After the second operation I felt much better, but I had to stay in the hospital for almost two months. During all that time I had a special duty nurse, very nice looking and very efficient, in her late twenties. I do not know how to say it, but I felt better when she was around, and only when she was around. She was like that not only with me but with all other patients, as I could see. When I was discharged, I needed some part-time nursing care at home where I was living alone, and I was glad to have her accept this job. I enjoyed her company tremendously and she stayed with me longer than required for my medical care. To make the story short; three months after my operation we were married, with my cardiologist's approval, although the doctor insisted that sex should be without stress.

It did not work too well. She turned out to be very passionate, in need of daily sex and I could not provide it more than once a week and even then she had to be in charge of all the mechanics of sexual activity, with me playing a passive role. I wanted her to quit her job but she did not want to. She loved her job, she said, and I can understand that. Two months ago she told me that she was involved in a sexual affair with a hospital employee. I do not know how to explain it, but I felt relief that somebody else was taking charge of her excessive passion. She would agree to whatever I wanted to do, although she maintained that she still loved me but in a different way. I also loved her in a different way and I was not ready to let her go.

We now have come to a silent agreement. I do not want to know what she does outside. Frankly, I do not mind at all being alone a few hours a day, while she is busy at her work or whatever. Otherwise we stay together with the same limited sexual activity. I do not know how long it will last but it is working. It may last for a while because, from what she tells me, her sexual "compensator" is married with two children, therefore not ready to divorce and take her away from me.

* * *

I am a 71 year old widow, still good looking, at least I think, and certainly still desirous for sex. My sexual desires are so intense that sometimes I pay gentlemen for favors. I finally arrived at a mode of living which I hope will be permanent at least for a while. I hired a South American fellow to do a painting job in my house. During his job I offered him breakfast and lunch and we talked. This is the usual method I follow to recruit a paid sexual partner. Anyway, this time it looked permanent. He was an illegal immigrant who came here on a student visa that has run out. I offered him marriage to legalize his immigration papers, and I will support him during his studies which may last a couple of years. We agreed on how much I will pay for his expenses and that we shall be 'intimate' about twice a week. He mentioned that he has a girlfriend also, which I did not care about, as long as he sticks to our agreement. This has been working well for the last five months. I can feel however that there is no love in his sex, although I reach climax most of the time, but I cannot require more than what I asked for. In the meantime, I returned to work on a part-time basis, commission only, in the real estate agency where I worked all my life.

Impotence and Frigidity

I am a 65 year old male. I married at the age of 24 and had two children, a boy and a girl. Sexual activity during my marriage was normal: two-to-three sexual acts a week, with my wife reaching orgasm most of the time. My marriage lasted 22 years. We started having arguments of increasing severity the last three years of our marriage. I learned later that my wife was having an affair with somebody and she went to live with him after we divorced. My two children were in college and their parents' divorce was not too traumatic for them. At least, I did not think so. Two years after the divorce I went to live with a woman about my age. Then I discovered to my dismay that I could not have an erection. For a few months I tried all kinds of medical and paramedical treatments with no success. My lady friend did not mind and would have liked to keep me as a companion. Besides I was expert in stimulating her clitoris and vagina to a sexual orgasm, which satisfied her entirely. But I became more and more uncomfortable with the whole thing and we split after one year. Lately, I even tried Viagra without any success. I am the director of a summer camp. Some of the camper's mothers are divorced and know of my divorced status (women always seem to know who are the divorced or widowed men), and occasionally made advances to me. I discouraged all of them because I never mixed my personal life with my business life, and because I was impotent. For the last 15 years I have lived alone and have not had any sexual relations during all that time.

Q. Do you have any desire for sexual activity?

A. Occasionally. But it does not last. About once a week I join a couple of widowed or divorced men who get together and watch sex movies while drinking beer.

Q. Do you have sexual fantasies?

A. Not often. They are initiated by the sex movies. They are no different from the sex movies.

Q. Do you have sexual dreams?

A. Very seldom. I do not remember any of them.

Q. Do you masturbate?

A. I tried for a while, but I cannot get any erection or ejaculation. I gave it up entirely.

Q. Is there any aspect of your current sexuality that we did not cover.

A. I am now well-adjusted to life with no sex. I consider sexual activity boring and not worth the effort. There is a time for everything and I do not now consider sex necessary for my life.

Q. Do you have any questions?

A. Well, if you hear of any cure for my impotence, let me know, I may try it.

Classically, the man has to perform. His concept of masculinity is at stake and on the line. He judges himself and thinks the world judges him according to the number of sexual acts he can perform every week, the hardness of his erect penis, the persistence of erection during the sexual act, the number of thrusts before ejaculation, the abundant ejaculation, and last but not least, the ability to elicit orgasm in the female partner. The more he can do all these things, the stronger and more virile he thinks he is. These concepts may appear grotesque but they are common especially in the young. Of course, as the young adult becomes older he learns better, namely that gentleness is more important than physical strength and rough sex, and that tender loving care is more meaningful in eliciting climax in the partner than anything else. He also may or may not learn to take part of the blame when sexual life is a failure.

The adult woman has a very different perspective during the sexual act. She can be completely passive, inert, and just let herself be penetrated: no exhausting physical motion, no hard erection to be maintained throughout, no tiring thrusts, no ejaculations to worry about. This ideal position is restful for the woman and many take advantage of it (Position #1, Table 22). My finding as an obstetrician and gynecologist involved in private practice and in hospital outpatient departments is that about 75% of adult female sexual activity is rather passive.

Of course not all female sexual acts are passive and many women have different attitudes. The woman may be on top and the roles are reversed (Position #2, Table 22), male passivity versus female activity. Most of all, many women are desirous of reaching orgasm and take an active role in its achievement, and may express concern in not being able to achieve it and being called frigid.

In summary there cannot be coitus with an impotent male, but there is possible coitus with a frigid female.

Let us now study how this sexual activity and passivity, how the fear of impotence and frigidity, are modified in seniors. We will see that the sexual fears of adult men diminish and even disappear or are magnified in seniors.

Progressive Diminution of Sexual Activity in Senior Age

The sexual behavior of seniors is determined by the following factors:

* The physical and/or mental illnesses which may impair or make impossible any sexual activity. A reservation has to be made about those physical illnesses that are treatable.
* A general weakness of the human body, which is more evident in the eighties and nineties and which could make difficult or even impossible the necessary effort for the sexual act. The active partner in the new sexual act, usually the male, would therefore be the first to become inactive.
* The interest in sexual activity which could decrease with advancing age, but really follows no rule. It may disappear early in senior age, may have disappeared even before senior age, or it may persist very late in age, even in the nineties. Some other subjects may even increase their sexual activity during their senior years explaining that they now have a lot of free time and have finished all obligations imposed on them during adult life.
* Men may be concerned about losing their libido, and may want to keep a macho attitude to hide impotence or fear of it. They may resort to a baculum insertion, to Viagra, or other techniques.
* Women may have a fear of no longer being attractive and will resort to excessive make-up, ostentatious jewelry or clothing, and finally plastic surgery all over the body (face, eyelids, neck, breast, abdomen, hips, and so on). Occasionally men resort to plastic surgery

too, such as hair transplants and liposuction.

* Men and more so women may be influenced in their sexual behavior by what I call outside factors, namely religious, moral, social, legal, and familial. Guilt feelings of getting involved sexually may be very strong among widows more than among widowers. The classic ascetic concept that sex is not to be practiced by seniors has to be overcome.

* Availability of a willing sexual partner is crucial in senior citizens even among married couples if one of the spouses is not sexually available. In this matter, senior women have a harder time than men first because there are more senior women than men and also women are (relatively) more inhibited in the search for a partner.

* Love is present among senior men and women, just as much as it is present among adults. It may be the same especially among couples that age together. However, just as often, the love feeling may change profoundly. Some couples, after liberation from all duties and obligations of the previous years, may love each other more as their relationship becomes more intense even if their sexual activity diminishes. Some others hold onto whatever relationship they had previously out of habit or inability to face major changes. For other couples, however, their differences, which were latent and hidden during their adulthood because of their familial and social obligations, now come to the open. Their common life, including their sexual life, is terminated.

Finally, among seniors there is an increasing desire to be liberated from any preconceived or pre-established ideas about their sexuality, a desire to explore it their own way without being told what to do and what not to do. There is a wish to discover, to make up a sexuality that is specifically suited to their own needs. A remark often made to me by some bitter women deprived of sex is the following: "It is acceptable for an old man to pay a young woman for sex. I know many seniors who do it and even brag about it. If I did the same with a young man, I would be ashamed and made fun of."

Evolution of the Species

In order to understand sexual evolution we have to go to basic trends in human behavior, namely human evolution. In his "Evolution of the Species," Charles Darwin has described what he calls natural selection and survival of the fittest. It goes this way. A given species is faced with an important change in the ecological environment, such as change in temperature, food supply, or invasion by a competing species. Most individuals in that species do not adapt to this change and will perish. Only those few individuals who present a specific adaptation to the change, such as thicker fur to protect against cold weather, or ability to adapt to a different food supply, or the capability of running away faster from a predator, or fight more strongly, etc., will survive. These new adaptees are the only ones to survive as individuals, but the only way they can survive as a species is by producing a progeny that will carry the new adaptation. The result is the permanent appearance of a new species presenting the new adaptation, while the original species disappears or survives only in an area that did not present any ecological change. This is how the various species evolve, presenting more and more adaptation to the environment and being more and more different from the original ones. This is what Charles Darwin called natural selection and survival of the fittest. Nature selects for survival and reproduction only those individuals that present adaptations necessary for survival in a constantly changing environment, eliminating all the misfits. Reproduction is what evolution is about because it is by successful transmission of the new adaptation to the progeny that evolution is successful. The strongest lion will secure and is attracted to the lionesses who produce the strongest pheromones, in order to satisfy his copulating needs that can be very high: almost every fifteen minutes during the peak season. Therefore, only the strongest males and only the females emitting the strongest pheromones will copulate and reproduce while the weaker individuals are pushed aside and most likely have no chance for copulation and no chance to reproduce and perpetuate their misfit condition. This is how each species maintains itself in excellent shape, continuously eliminating the misfits, and keeping itself as a 'pure' species.

At the time the current Homo sapiens appeared, his life span rarely extended beyond 40 years, and it remained more or less the same until a century ago. All individuals were on top of their physical and sexual performance until the end of their life which, I repeat, was in the early forties. Then around 40 years of age, there was a rapid decline and death. Men died of accidents, women in childbirth, and everybody died also of malnutrition, starvation, and infection (mostly pneumonia and bronchopneumonia). From the earliest form of the prehuman species of two million years ago, up to the present Homo sapiens who appeared about forty thousand years ago, the fittest for survival and for reproduction were progressively selected through elimination of the less fit. Natural selection has done an excellent job for human sexuality in terms of selecting the fittest for reproduction. From the beginning of mankind the strongest and the most intelligent individuals were mating with the most beautiful and healthiest women. We now have a strong definition of nature, of what is natural. Is natural what has been naturally selected by survival of the fittest and elimination of the misfits.

Reproductive Organs or Sexual Organs

Why do we get involved in sexual activity? What determines sexuality in general? For animals, the answer is very simple (Table 48). They copulate in order to reproduce. Even in animals this answer is not that simple however. For instance the above statement: "animals copulate in order to reproduce" is incorrect because animals have no idea whatsoever that copulation leads to reproduction. The whole coital and reproductive mechanism in animals is purely biological with no willful interference whatsoever and without the animal having any knowledge of reproduction.

I maintain that sex is not a pleasure in animals. In the male, there is only an urgent need to evacuate painfully distended seminal vesicles. In the female it is estrus or heat, i.e., it is an inflamed and painful organ. Animal sex and reproduction are purely biological.

The great difference between animal and human sexuality is that animal sexuality is purely and solely a contact between sexual organs of the opposite sex (Table 48). Humans also establish sexual contact like animals, but they also have the opportunity to establish contact between two individuals, body and soul. Animals only copulate, while humans copulate and relate. On purpose I say 'copulate' first and 'relate' second, because more often than not the human sexual relation turns out to be only for copulation. On the contrary, seniors have the opportunity to 'relate' first and 'copulate' second, and they can even relate and not copulate at all.

Many biologists call the human genitals the reproductive organs and do not distinguish human sex from human reproduction. This may be true for animals where sexual activity is solely geared toward reproduction, but not so in humans where reproduction and sex are completely separate from one another. Among the large number of sexual acts that men and women are involved in during their lifetime, one may wonder how many are directed toward reproduction. Barely any. In this study let us separate human sexuality from human reproduction and investigate them separately. This separation will be important when we differentiate senior and adult human sexuality.

Let us start with sex (Table 48). There are fundamental differences between human and animal sex. Human sexuality is still biological but to a small degree. Sexual hormones are still present but in no way entirely determine human sex. Estrus in the female is barely noticeable, if at all; pheromones have disappeared and there is no longer olfactory stimulation in the male. No one has ever proven that sexual activity is determined by the level of sexual hormones (estrogen, testosterone) in the body. Estrogen intake does not cure a woman's frigidity or increase her sex activity any more than testosterone intake cures a man's impotence or increases male sexual desire.

A little known human phenomenon is that during orgasm there is no increase whatsoever in the estrogen level in females or the testosterone level in males (Mature Sexuality, Patient Realities and Provider Challenges, Clinical Proceedings, Sept. 2000)). This is so different from animals where testosterone in males and estrogen in females determine the whole coital behavior; in animals outside of the heat period, these levels are low and at that time there is no sexual activity of any kind. Why did the sexual (really reproductive) hormones stop playing a fundamental role in human sexuality? The reason for this is the tremendous enlargement of the human brain which has taken over and now interferes with and even determines many body functions. Specifically, sexual activity, purely hormonal in animals, has become much less hormonal and essentially cerebral in humans. The cerebral influence can be mental or emotional, conscious or unconscious, it does not matter. The simplistic animal sexuality has become much more complex in humans in view of these cerebral interferences. In all of my various research programs, I have constantly stressed that the main difference between animal and human sexuality is that the former is purely hormonal and is initiated by pheromones the pathway of which is olfactory, while the latter is mostly neurological and cerebral, the pathway of which is visual and tactile. To put it in different words, animals sniff sex while humans see it, touch it, hear of it, think of it. Women do anything they can to reactivate the prehuman olfactory aspect of sex through the use of perfumes, but this is of limited effect because the part of the brain reserved to olfaction is limited in humans while the visual, tactile, and auditory are predominant. Figure 11 shows the animal brain and Figure 12 shows the human brain and the olfactory zones are compared showing the relatively large olfactory zone in animals and the small one in humans.

Let us go now to the reproductive function in humans. It remains purely biological and hormonal just like in animals. The biology of human pregnancy is identical to animals. It is essentially regulated by estrogen and progesterone that are produced in large quantity by the ovaries and the placenta.

The above physiological data, although possibly arduous to follow, are crucial for understanding sexuality in the senior community. Women go through menopause, their ovaries become atrophic and no longer produce estrogen. In the male climacteric, the testes produce less and less testosterone. Whatever limited role is left for reproductive hormones in human adult life, it completely ceases in senior life. For those who want to argue about the role of reproductive hormones in human sex, this argument ceases for senior citizens. There are no more reproductive hormones to play a role in senior sexual life. Senior sexuality is not based on any hormones whatsoever. The presence of sexual activity in seniors is the best proof that it is not based on the presence of sexual hormones. The administration of sexual hormones to humans of any age has very limited medical indications (and is associated with serious side effects) that have absolutely nothing to do with sexuality and never produce sexual stimulation.

We can now summarize the scientific aspects of human sexuality, as drawn from the above research, by saying that senior sexuality is not geared toward reproduction, since both males and females have passed the reproductive age, and is not determined by reproductive hormones, since the levels of these hormones are very low. Therefore, senior sexuality is a purely cerebral and mental phenomenon. This conclusion is crucial in understanding senior sexuality.

Other consequences can be drawn from the above conclusions. Or, rather, important questions are raised. Once we eliminated biological (hormonal) drive and reproductive function, then why sex in seniors? Is it necessary, is it healthy, or is it stressful and harmful? Does it have any other function, so far unsuspected? Should it be discouraged in those who practice it, or encouraged in those who feel inhibited indulging in it? Of course there is no single answer to the above problems, and as we have seen in the interviews, the approach to these problems are multiple depending on the senior individual.

Change in Sexual Posture

At the dawn of mankind sexual behavior could be reconstructed as follows. Early male hominids (between apes and humans) had no reason or desire to change their animal ancestry as far as sex was concerned. These 'animal-men' penetrated the female from behind just like the mounting position in animals. This position was very uncomfortable for the primitive human female who was getting more and more acquainted with erect posture. As much as she could, very patiently over millions of years, the female requested 'face-to-face' posture for coitus, most likely with a not very cooperative male, but the woman more and more persistent.

Once the face-to-face position became the rule, the sexual partners could look at and start to recognize each other. At this stage the primitive human female was in a difficult quandary. Because of all the anatomical changes associated with erect posture the female was very reluctant to assume the quadrupedal posture necessary for male mounting because it was uncomfortable and even painful. This primitive female started to prefer lying on her back and spreading her knees for coitus, while the primitive man did not see any reason to change anything and resisted changing positions. How this sexual drama got resolved over millions of years is hard to understand, but not so difficult to imagine. The human female prevailed and the mounting position was completely given up and replaced by other positions. Let us notice that there are casual returns to animal posture since our animal ancestry is only skin deep. The current prevailing one is the woman lying rather passively on her back and the man being in charge of most of the sexual activity. Regardless of the claims by numerous biologists, this new sexual posture is unique to humans. For the first time during the billions of years of history of life on earth, sexual posture has changed.

This new posture had tremendous advantages for the female. It is more restful than the mounting position and she is more in control of the sexual act since it is rather difficult to make her spread her legs unless she cooperates. Most of all, she identifies the sexual partner, or rather the two sexual partners easily identify each other first during coitus then outside of it. Now in the face-to-face posture, the two partners can look fully at each other and all their emotions are exposed: pain, fear, hate, indifference, comfort, pleasure, and soon love. This is completely novel in the evolution of the species and opens the door to the fact that human evolution may be nothing else but sexual evolution.

As our primitive ancestors became more intelligent (Homo erectus, the Neanderthals, Archaic Homo sapiens), they tended to form primitive social nuclei. Emotions and love became more involved with the sexual act. Besides, primitive women had more difficulties during pregnancy especially late in pregnancy, more difficulties during labor and delivery, and more involvement in the newborn, which of all mammals is the most helpless during the first years of life. The family unit was born. Once the male discovered that coitus led to impregnation, a very late knowledge in human history since even today some primitive societies in remote parts of the world do not have that knowledge and consider pregnancy a magic event, the family unit took a final form. The male was the head of the family who put his seed in the female womb; he was the real father of his children, he was a responsible provider. The woman was responsible for the children and preparation of food and could be a food gatherer collecting grains and fruits. She was also available for the sexual needs of the head of the family unit. The woman needed a responsible man for continuing protection and as a food provider. She progressively lost her estrus or sexual swelling of her genital area because she wanted to be sexually available solely to one man, and not a mob of sexually stimulated men. Today we call it concealed estrus, but truly it is almost all gone. As the children grew up and reached puberty, they left the family unit; the boys left on their own or were expelled and the girls were taken or given as sexual partners to start a new family unit.

The important aspect of this original family unit was that for practical purposes the women were either pregnant or nursing (which usually inhibits menstrual periods). The result was that women almost never had menstrual periods since they quickly passed from puberty to pregnancy to nursing, then pregnancy again, and so on. Women (and men for that matter) never reached menopause since death in their thirties and rarely in their early forties, was the rule. It might have taken one to two hundred thousand years for this primitive family pattern to become firmly established, and until recently it was modified only in details varying from one culture to another. The basic aspects have barely changed: the man is a responsible food provider and protector and the mother gives birth to children and raises them. From the sexual point of view the man learned to be faithful to the family unit although outside indulgences and even polygamy were frequent. Let us stress that if the concept of the family unit was not created, the survival of the human culture as it is today would have been impossible because the woman was physically weaker and needed a reliable and constant protector and provider during pregnancy, childbirth, nursing and all other aspects of her life. The social structure, law, religion, customs, all stepped in to reinforce the ties of the original family unit. Man and woman became husband and wife permanently united and more or less faithful to each other, and responsibility for their children became consecrated until the children became adults.

In order to reinforce this family unit, emotional attachment and love for each other was on the rise: love of the mother for her children which extended beyond the biological attachment of animals where the maternal care for the animal newborn and infant almost always ceases with the end of nursing, with return of estrus and with the next pregnancy. This new human mother was really attached to all her children acquired during successive pregnancies; love of the father for his children who were the product of his own seed; most of all, love between men and women, both looking at each other during sex, then between sex, and thus reaching the stars. Sadness and sorrow were also acquired as parents lost a large number of their children in childbirth or in infancy, as women died in childbirth (the most common cause of death in women), as men died from wounds and infections following hunting and tribal wars.

Mind and Sex

If one wants to speak about our animal ancestry, the animal sexual attraction has completely disappeared in humans. No matter what the pseudo-science claims are, there is no return to animal pheromones and there is not even space in the human brain to respond to any sexual stimulation of olfactory origin. Comparatively speaking, the olfactory zone is much smaller in the human than in the animal brain (Figure 11). What now makes sexual attraction in humans is completely different. Human sexual attraction is essentially visual and tactile. Animal males do not pay attention to the visual appearance of the female and there is barely any touching in animal sex except between the genital organs.

Visual identification of the sexual partner is a human acquisition and tactile stimulation or sex stimulation by touch is also a human acquisition. In addition, the human attraction is very individual and only to a specific partner. Although I do not deny a limited biological or hormonal role in human sexuality, the attraction is still essentially mental. In humans it is a visual and also tactile stimulus that is transmitted to the brain; then the brain stimulates the human genital organs and produces a desire for copulation. These different pathways are essential to understand, to study human and senior sexuality.

The visual identification of the human sexual partner leads to a new feeling for that specific individual, and an emotional attachment and love for that partner and no other since the sexual partner can now be visually recognized. One could argue, specifically on the male side, that coitus can also be casual. But even so, such as the case of a female prostitute for instance, there is some visual selection of the partner. A sexual act is the expression of a relationship rather than an end to itself. It is never a purely biological phenomenon. Whenever I hear a man brag about the last female prostitute he just met, I push the conversation to the point of exasperation by asking him to describe the physical appearance of the prostitute, what he liked in her, would he like to see her again, how he feels about her, any detail about her private life, and so on. Humans want to know whom they have sex with, not animals. Human sex is highly individualized. This is the fundamental characteristic of human sex and the main difference with animal sex.

In this respect, women are much more advanced than men. No woman gets involved sexually unless and until she really knows whom she is getting involved with. The only exception is the prostitute and even in this case, there is often a pimp behind or she does it for money. When an emotional relationship is pushed to the extreme, it becomes love, and sexual desire is preferentially directed to a specifically loved partner.

Sexual activity in the 60s, 70s, and 80s with complete orgasm while the testes and ovaries are completely atretic and non-functional is the very proof that human sex is mostly and essentially a cerebral (mental and emotional) phenomenon. It is mostly in the mind. This is the reason why mentally retarded people have limited or no sexuality. Of course the fact that the mind alone has the sexual field for itself and is left alone to deal with sexuality, especially with a progressively weaker and more handicapped body, produces specific characteristics and a tremendous variety in senior sexuality. Specifically there may be a discrepancy between a persistent or even increased sexual desire and a weaker body that limits the physical effort necessary for sexual performance, especially in males. Basically, the sexual desire may be limited, or if still present the senior body may perform differently or may need extra help that we will detail later. But the classic concept that there should be no senior sex because biological hormones and reproduction are gone, has no basis whatsoever. The mind of the senior citizen can still be intact and that is all that is needed to carry on sexually (Tables 43-46).

Anatomical Differences and Sexual Repercussions

A question that has intrigued researchers on human sexuality is the following. Why is it that men run after women for sex and not the opposite? Why is sex, in general, a favor women granted to men and not the opposite? The above data provides the answer: it is a question of supply and demand. There are more men than women looking for sex, or, rather, men look for sex more frequently than women. Men are sexually stimulated much more frequently than women. This makes women more desirable and men run after them. This also explains why men have sex with different partners more often than women if we exclude prostitutes. The regular partner may not be available as often as requested. Women look for intimacy in sex more than men and have a tendency to stick with a single partner more often.

That men look for sexual activity much more than women has been shown by many authors: Kinsey, et al. have statistically investigated how often men, compared to women, look for coitus, how many times a day or a week they indulge in it, how many different partners they get involved with successively or concomitantly. It is also a fact that men spend little time in foreplay and go directly for vaginal penetration. Men usually can wait a relatively short period of time (a few weeks at most) between two sexual acts and have a tendency to look for another partner beside the regular one if the latter is not available, while women can go for much longer periods of sexual abstention (see Table 29). Men have a tendency to consider that coitus is terminated immediately after ejaculation while women would like to keep the romance going even after the male partner withdraws (Table 23). Men have a tendency to think of sex as an interaction between two opposite sex organs, while women would rather look at it as an interaction between two entire bodies and souls, between two total individuals. There are houses of prostitution and female prostitutes to satisfy the additional male needs and there never has been houses of prostitution for additional sexual female needs. The list can be extended indefinitely, although I will not deny that each item can be argued, as there are numerous exceptions. The general tendency, however, is that men look for sex much more than women.

In the present chapter I will try to delve into what I think are the causes of these differences between male and female sexuality. This is crucial because the persistence or non-persistence of these causes (at least for some), will be of tremendous help in understanding sexuality during senior age.

Let us start with the evolutionary point of view. When a man is described as behaving 'like an animal,' this description is often correct because this is how practically all animals behave. The strongest animal male surrounds himself with as many females as he can control and indulges himself continuously from a coital point of view. The animal female has little say in the matter. Some biologists have described isolated animal species as 'pairing.' This 'pairing' is rare, more apparent than real, and not sexual anyway. Assuming that animal ancestry leaves an imprint in human males and in some way it certainly does, then we have a 'hereditary base' for such remnants of animal behavior in human males.

Next, I have an important list of anatomical considerations that could account for more sexual drive in men than in women. Male genitals (penis and scrotum containing the testicles) are exposed externally and are continuously touched, massaged, etc. Quite often the skin of the penis and scrotum is stuck at the inner thighs in an embarrassing manner. None of these anatomical and physiological considerations exist in females since there is no emission of any fluid content through the female urethra during climax, and no penis or scrotum to hang between upper inner thighs. The tremendous differences between males and females in anatomy of the sex organs and physiology of coitus are such that the male has to be active and ejaculate for proper sexual activity, while the female has a choice: she can also be active but just as often the female can be passive, non-participating, or even partially or totally frigid during coitus.

These are other major differences between men and women that have an effect on sexual stimulation. The main erotic parts of the female body, namely the clitoris and the vaginal entrance, are essentially concealed within the female body. Even the nipples are well protected under a bra away from any constant rubbing. On the contrary, the erotic zones of the male body, namely penis and scrotum, are being constantly rubbed against each other, against the inner thighs, against clothing, and even when sleeping and constantly changing positions when in bed. It is unbelievable how much and how often the male organs are touched and stimulated during sleep. It is not very intense but it can go on for hours. It is equivalent to a "mini" masturbation and it is no wonder men often wake up in the middle of the night in full erection.

Finally, from the biological point of view, ovaries cease to function in women at menopause around the age of 50, and therefore no longer produce estrogen; while the testes keep functioning and producing sperm and testosterone in advanced age (although to a lesser degree), thus making the man capable of filling his seminal vesicles and creating the need for their evacuation through orgasm and ejaculation. The man can also be capable of fertilizing and be sexually potent at a very advanced age. Male climacteric (or male menopause) occurs much later in life and is not always total.

There are also physiological differences that result in additional sexual stimulations in the male. When the male urinary bladder is full, it presses on the prostate and seminal vesicles. And when the urinary bladder is full, the internal sphincter opens up, this resulting in the urge for urination and also sexual stimulation since the upper urethral canal is erotogenic. Therefore, when the bladder fills up during sleep, it frequently leads to male erection, which is relieved only after urination. Finally, the whole urethral mucosa is erotogenic and urination by itself is sexually stimulating in a mild way. There is an intimate association between sex and urination since ejaculation of sperm through the urethra leads to male orgasm. Let us add that during urination, the penis is extensively manipulated to hold steady the urinary stream and this also adds an opportunity for sex stimulation.

Women are completely deprived of (or I should say spared) all these stimulations of tactile and urinary origin, which, in view of their frequency lead the male to constant sexual stimulation. It is no wonder that men look for sex much more often than women.

The above anatomy and physiology does not explain all the differences between male and female human sexuality. There is human culture, which as far back as one can go has always been directed toward sexual indulgence in men and sexual inhibition in women. There certainly are other differences of emotional and mental origin, but the role of those above, too often ignored, deserves to be listed. The grotesque and clownish role of the man conquering a woman even when he has no real sexual desire is not to be overlooked. One should not forget that sexual advertising of any and all kinds is always directed toward male stimulation and almost never toward female stimulation. This is the very proof that males are more sexually responsive than females.

The result of all the above differences is that males are constantly stimulated, sexually speaking, while females are much less. When society requires that we control our sexual drives or instincts, it is much easier for women than for men to follow the rule and do so. In fact, biologists talk often about 'concealed estrus' in women. I would rather call it markedly weakened or even absent estrus. Not being preoccupied in being sexually *stimulated* as much as men, women can concentrate on what they can do best, that is sexually *stimulating* men mainly through their visual appearance or beauty. This is the present picture of our current society: stimulated men and stimulating women. Social rules are rather harsh for men who cannot control these constant sexual stimulations, and are rather liberal for women who, in the name of freedom of expression, are continuously stimulating. If men controlled their sexual drives the way women do, human sexuality and the human species would be markedly altered and even in danger of disappearing. If men were not sexually stimulated more than women, and if they diminished their sexual interest, the whole human culture would be in jeopardy. This is partially happening with the spread of homosexuality and less heterosexual marriages.

For some of the women who still have some sexual drives that cannot be concealed or that cannot be satisfied with hetero- or homosexuality, there is masturbation. Masturbation is a general phenomenon among women and it is active from early infanthood to the most advanced age. Most masturbating women can reach climax. They reach masturbating orgasm easily because they have all the time and patience to learn how to do it, they do it only when in the mood to indulge in it, without waiting for a male partner who may have his own sexual schedule. It is very easy for a female to discover the clitoris and the vaginal entrance as being erotic zones during her body exploration while washing herself or putting on clothes. Since she is told early in life by her family, by religious authorities, and by society in general that this is condemned she keeps it to herself and does not even tell her intimate friends. All it takes is a few strokes with a finger around the genitals for a minute or two and she gets her orgasm. She can do it while taking a shower or a bath, or before going to sleep. For those females who have scruples of any kind in using their fingers, they can use any object, rub against panties, or rub their thighs against each other, or while using soap, and it is not masturbation anymore! Modern women even use vibrators or other more specialized tools. Women can do it on a daily or monthly basis, even when married. It is in masturbation that most women first discover climax and later on try to extend it in heterosexuality. Some women succeed in using masturbation as a preparation to heterosexuality, but some do not make the transfer and are content with masturbation. Some women use preparatory masturbation prior to heterosexual orgasm when the male partner is rushing his own orgasm. When the male has reached his orgasm and leaves the female partner unsatisfied, she may go to the bathroom to masturbate until satisfied. If women do not find any or enough orgasms in heterosexuality, they can always find it in masturbation. Not all women masturbate but almost half of them do.

Men also masturbate mostly during adolescence, but they have a tendency to diminish it or even give it up as they advance in age. There is some kind of taboo against male masturbation. It is almost an evidence that one is unable to find and seduce a female partner, i.e., a sign of incompetence and even impotence. There is a noticeable difference between boys and girls as far as the beginning of masturbation is concerned. In boys, it is a volitional act needing planning and it is a noticeable activity. Boys have to go through an elaborate preparation in order to masturbate and there is always ejaculation, a physical proof of masturbation. Boys often do it in groups. In girls and adolescent women, it can occur spontaneously, or during activities like bicycling, any sport, or taking a shower. It is always done privately. The physical activity leading to female masturbation is rather minimal.

The History of Sexual Stimulation

One may wonder why sexual stimulation is the greatest satisfaction and pleasure in humans. The origin is biological and evolutionary in nature. To begin with, one can observe in the animal world how much skin contact is pleasurable. Such isolated examples of pleasurable touching in animals can be observed in nature. Bears find tremendous pleasure in romping. All primates spend as much time in grooming each other as looking for food. Animals constantly lick each other. When one observes a group of lions at rest, they practically always sleep on top of each other. The art of domesticating animals is very simple, and it essentially consists in touching the animals as much as possible. To touch a horse, an elephant, a parakeet, is knowing how much they enjoy being touched and knowing how to touch them. A cat or a dog will constantly look to be touched more than anything else, even more than being fed.

But the main difference between animals and humans is the skin. All animals have a skin thickly covered with hair to protect them against cold weather and to act as a shield against trauma. This makes skin contact difficult and limited. The main exception is the mother animal who immediately after giving birth indulges in thoroughly licking her litter. Then during the whole nursing period, her nipples become a source of constant contact stimulation.

Finally, contact with genital organs is stimulating. In order to maintain reproduction, nature (or evolution) has made the genital organs covered with a tremendous amount of nervous endings, thus making their contact very stimulating, i.e., sexually stimulating. The genital organs of male and female are tremendously congested during the "heat" season and therefore more responsive to contact stimulation.

Sexually stimulated animals could indulge in masturbation, but they have no hands except for primates. So, some animals will rub their genitals against any object, such as a branch or the trunk of a tree, a stone, or anything else. Primates have hands and they frequently indulge in masturbation when no female is around or when displaced from available female by superior hierarchy. At any rate, masturbation is much less frequent in animals than reported by superficial observers. Animals, specifically primates, take all kinds of postures and touch themselves and each other all over their body indiscriminately, thus taking certain postures or making certain actions that may appear sexual but really are not.

In light of the evolutionary review, where do humans stand? First, practically the whole human body becomes erotogenic because, except for part of the head covered by hair the whole human skin is naked and therefore exposed and responsive to contact and stimulation. Some parts of the human skin are more erogenous than others depending on individuals. In the human female, the nipples, the clitoris, and the vaginal entrance are specifically erogenous. In the male, the penis and the skin covering the testicles are erogenous. In both men and women the anal entrance could also be erogenous.

Second, humans are stimulated all year round and not only during the "heat" season. The seasonal pheromones, which are powerful sexual stimuli in animals, have disappeared in humans, and are replaced in humans by tactile, visual (beauty), auditory, or mental stimuli which are constantly available. It is true that these new stimuli are not as powerful as the pheromones, but they are perennial, and not seasonal. Therefore, humans are sexually stimulated all year around from puberty on, and even before puberty.

Third, Homo sapiens, or wise man, is a thinking man or woman, with the ability to think, reflect, ponder on his/her actions. Specifically, human sexual drives are under conscious control. To put it differently, humans are supposed to control their sexual instincts and not submit to them nor follow them entirely the way animals do. They can sexually stimulate themselves, without any outside stimulus. It is mostly through control of sexual drive that human society became possible.

The Discovery of Orgasm in Humans

This discovery is rather autoerotic in the human species.

In the male, as explained previously, erection occurs at any age after birth in view of the 'external' exposure and continuous stimulation of the penis and scrotum. It is only in puberty that the juvenile is exposed to full orgasm with ejaculation in erotic dreams and/or masturbation. It is secondarily, by being visually exposed to females, that the male discovers that the whole gamut of orgasm (i.e. erection, coitus and ejaculation) is made more satisfactory and pleasurable in heterosexuality than in autoeroticism and masturbation.

The female more or less goes through a similar cycle. She also discovers sexual stimulation of her clitoris and vaginal entrance early in life either with her fingers or using any object. Also, at puberty, she discovers full orgasm in erotic dreams and/or full masturbation. Finally she discovers heterosexual orgasm. Opposite to men who realize heterosexual orgasm early in life, women acquire it progressively and more slowly, if at all. They have to overcome inhibitions.

There is however a crucial difference between the young male and female in terms of sexual orgasm. The young male has relatively minimal difficulty in the transition from autoeroticism to heterosexuality. Heterosexuality comes rather naturally and he easily transfers from nocturnal ejaculation and masturbation to coitus, without necessarily giving up entirely nocturnal ejaculation and/or masturbation as such. Maladjustments in males are not frequent and rather easy to overcome, and the enjoyments of heterosexuality by petting and/or coitus become predominant. The young female on the contrary has more difficulty and takes more time in the transition. In fact some women never make the full transition and never experience orgasm in coitus, or experience it infrequently and/or incompletely. While the first coitus in males is easy and looked forward to and usually immediately successful, it is completely different in the virginal female. There is fear of losing her virginity (a high social status), fear of the defloration being painful, fear of the unknown, fear of pregnancy, fear of breaking social, cultural, religious, or moral taboos. It is a common and ordinary knowledge among pubescent and teenage girls that the purpose of the first sexual act or acts is not so much orgasm, but defloration, or breaking through the hymen, which can be painful and is approached with much apprehension. It is only later on, with more coital experience that orgasm in females becomes established, hopefully.

To further complicate the situation in the new woman (and by 'new,' I mean new in terms of coitus), she is rather highly individual in her choice of a male partner. An adolescent man is not necessarily selective in choosing his first female partner. He is not necessarily selective in his first choice since he is looking as much for anonymous heterosexual orgasm as for orgasm with a specific female selected well in advance, and a prostitute will usually do. I know quite a few adolescent men who have a 'steady' girlfriend with whom sex is limited to petting for the time being and with whom they have future plans, but have another girlfriend or prostitutes on the side that are used solely for full coitus with orgasm and ejaculation. Adolescent females rarely do it on the first date, and then only after much petting, hesitation, resistance, and usually with the same boyfriend/partner. Of course there are many variations especially with the new generation.

We now can perceive the sexual difference between animals and humans. In humans, something has been added to the biological animal. True, there are still biological imperatives in humans, but they are not sexual imperatives and are no longer dominant. A man and a woman, each one with specific values, face each other, unite with each other, clash against each other, try to perceive each other and perceive the universe beyond their biological origins, and unfortunately too often fail to do so. Coitus may be an end to itself in humans as it is in animals, but the potential union of the two sexual partners that goes beyond sexual coitus is always there.

There are still some animal remnants in human sexuality: violence, rape, aggression, hierarchy (dominant males acquiring as many females as they can handle, thus depriving the average male of any sexual outlet), and complete submission of the abused females. These laws of nature are only skin deep in humans, especially in males. Therefore moral behavior, ethics, culture, customs, law, society, all step in to regulate this potential chaos, which, if left uncontrolled, would make human society impossible.

We can now summarize the different factors that determine human sexual behavior: reproduction and biological impulses, which are animal in origin; social regulations and ultimate transcendence to love, which are human additions. Orgasm is an enhanced quality of sex, and is specific to humans. How these different factors are affected in seniors will now be considered. Reproduction and biological drives are terminated with menopause in women and climacteric in men. Social regulations of all kinds, the purpose of which is to protect the social order and family unit are to be reconsidered since family responsibilities are over and seniors rarely disturb the social structure. What is left is the union and intimacy created by a communal life that many use but not necessarily use the previously inherited sexual patterns.

Students of female sexuality and women themselves

are often surprised at how easily a woman can reach orgasm through masturbation and yet often find it difficult and even impossible to reach during coitus. The reason is very simple. A woman masturbates only if she is mentally as well as physically ready. Masturbation is autoerotic and she knows very well how to stimulate herself, and does it at the appropriate time. If she is not ready, she just does not do it or does not finish it. In coitus she responds to another person who may make a sexual demand at a time when she is not in the mood (women can be moody, sexually and otherwise), who may not know how to arouse her the way she does with masturbation, or to spend the necessary time on it, or refuses to cooperate. This is the reason masturbatory orgasm is easier than coital orgasm. Not all mothers, not all husbands, know about the degree of masturbation in their daughters or spouses. The final aspect of masturbatory orgasm is that it is not as powerful as coital orgasm, for the simple reason that auto-satisfaction is not as powerful as hetero-satisfaction. It is an aspect of human nature that when two humans unite in a satisfactory act, their union adds a new dimension. Love between two people is more powerful than self love. Masturbatory orgasm is a 'local' and personal affair in the female (and male) body, but coital orgasm involves the whole mind and body of two separate individuals, and could become transcendent. When two humans of opposite sex become transcendent, they can reach the stars. Isolation leads some senior women to return (or discover) masturbation.

Sex in the Beginning

Is sex for pleasure or reproduction? Do we have sex organs or reproductive organs? Are estrogen and testosterone sexual hormones or reproductive hormones? It is still an unanswered problem, religiously, as well as scientifically. In order to clarity this problem, it is necessary to look at it from an evolutionary and historical point of view. The evolutionary point of view has already been covered; let us now cover the historical.

Adam and Eve were certainly attributed sex by God as a pure pleasure and for them, in the beginning at least, there was no question of reproduction. It is only after the incident of the forbidden fruit that reproduction and painful birth came about.

Early Christianity had a strict attitude toward sex and usually condemned it. For early Christians, sexual pleasure or what they called carnal satisfaction was associated with the numerous orgies so common during the decadence of the Roman Empire. They believed that passing through earthly life was an imposition and a constant temptation to sinful sex. There is happiness only when we join God. They did not believe that much in procreation, which would bring only more misery and more sins. Better to be married to God or join Him in heaven. The ecstasy of being with God is far beyond the earthly pleasure of sex. Sexual climax was not acceptable in Christianity. Therefore, there was not much room for sex of any kind in Christian life, and originally celibacy was preferred. It was only when they realized that total and general abstinence was impractical, not advisable because sinners would dominate the earth, and it was impossible to eradicate sex, that they limited celibacy to the clergy only. This has been maintained up to the present time although not as strictly. This is now called the Judeo-Christian tradition because traditional Judaism also frowns upon sexual pleasure. The only difference between traditional Judaism and early Christianity is that Judaism recognizes that it is impossible and not even desirable to resist the sexual drive and, anyway, sex is necessary for reproduction, which Judaism strongly encourages.

There was some return to pleasurable sex in the Christian world during the Renaissance, but the Reformed Church, after breaking with Roman Catholicism, essentially returned to an ascetic concept of sex, which was to be practiced only in marriage and even then for reproductive purposes only. The biologic aspect of sexuality was recognized to be much more accentuated in men who have a need for ejaculation than in women who are supposed to, and effectively do, completely inhibit their estrus. The biological drive was considered primitive behavior not worth any consideration from a religious man.

The classic and current attitude toward sex in the western culture is the Judeo-Christian tradition, namely that it is reserved for married people and only for reproductive purposes. From the religious, moral, legal, social, ethical, and familial point of view there is no sex for adolescent, single, widows and widowers, and most of all for post-menopausal women and post-climacteric men even if still married. Masturbation and homosexuality, which do not include procreation, are out of the question. This ascetic attitude, although consecrated by the powerful church and by law, was rarely followed by anyone at least not in the open. As we can see, humans are asked to be responsible for their sexual behavior and are supposed to entirely control it. An irresistible biological drive, as in animals, is not acceptable. The hazard of sex was always pregnancy, which, all too often was the responsibility of the woman. Up to the middle of the last century birth control was barely known and awkwardly practiced: withdrawal before ejaculation which supposes a concerned and cooperative male, or an immediate vaginal douche after ejaculation. Barely anybody adhered to these techniques, and up to a generation ago many marriages occurred because the future bride was already pregnant. An important breakthrough occurred with the more widespread practice of birth control, which allowed sex and avoided reproduction. For the first time in human history, starting in the first half of the 20th century, sex and reproduction could be separated. As birth control made tremendous progress, Roman Catholicism (and also Orthodox Judaism) were still opposed to any form of birth control and also to termination of pregnancy.

During the 20th century, especially the second half, a re-evaluation of the ascetic attitude took place progressively, and it became recognized that sex could be pleasurable by itself and not necessarily geared solely toward reproduction. It should be emphasized that restriction in sexual activity was a purely western occidental concept barely known in the rest of the world.

Earlier in the previous century as the number of seniors grew slowly and progressively, the classic opinion still was that there was no sex for them since they passed the age of reproduction. Seniors should have nothing to do with sex. Sexual unfaithfulness among adults could pass unnoticed, but the same event in people advanced in age would be considered scandalous.

One can see, as the senior population increased, seniors found themselves faced with a pattern of sexual behavior written especially for them by others and which was total abstinence, or at most limited sexuality for the 'younger' seniors that were still married.

A revolution in senior sexuality is in the offing.

The Ultimate Meaning of Sex

The above review of human sexuality, and its culmination in male orgasm and female climax, would be incomplete unless one ponders on the ultimate meaning of sex, and how it evolved from the animal condition. This question is very important because many researchers, including the most respected ones, have a tendency to equate animal and human sexuality. After all, the same organs and the same mechanics are involved, so why should the function be different? Many highly respected scientific authorities deny any difference.

Sexuality in animals, and I prefer the term copulation, is very simple. It has been previously described in detail and is summarized here. Biological hormones entirely control the mechanism of copulation. Castration in animals, i.e. removal of ovaries or testes, makes the animal completely asexual but hormonal injections reestablish copulation. Therefore, sexuality in animals is purely biological. There is no menopause or climacteric in animals and they are sexually active and reproductive all their life.

In humans there are different purposes in sexuality. True, they reproduce and sexuality is necessary for reproduction, but reproduction barely enters into play during sexuality. Hormones play a minimal role in human sexuality since castration barely alters it, and hormonal injections do not modify it. Besides, post-menopausal and post-climacteric senior citizens can have normal sexual activity with orgasm and climax. Therefore, sexuality in addition to being necessary for reproduction as it is in animal ancestry has found new goals in humans, namely sexual pleasure (orgasm and climax) and creation of intimacy between individuals of opposite gender.

The above reviews on animal and human sexuality are important if one is to understand and explore sexuality in seniors. It is only after considering human sexuality in adults and adolescents that one can get an idea on what basis to build senior sexuality. Is senior sexuality to be given up entirely or is it going to be similar to or different from adult sexuality? Is it going to reject it all together and build a new one on a different basis? Is it going to keep some part of it? We will attempt to answer some of these questions.

The History of Male Superiority in Sexuality

There is a traditional concept that in sexual activity, the male is the one who chooses the female partner, who initiates the sexual act, who determines how it should be performed, who decides when it should terminate, and in general who is the 'boss'. In all these activities the female partner traditionally is submissive, passive, and inactive. There are even some cultures where any active participation on the part of the woman in coitus is considered an intrusion on her part into the masculinity of the male. In some religious sects, it is bad tone for the female partner to be anything but immobile during coitus, and it is considered improper to move during the whole sexual process, or to initiate it an any way. Of course during history and in different cultures women have always found ways of initiating, directing, participating, even terminating the sexual act. How did this male superiority come about? In order to understand the problem, we have to go back again to our animal ancestry since numerous aspects of human sexuality show remnants of animal sexuality.

During the mating season (rams or sea lions) or all year round (lions, primates), the strongest male secures as many females around him as he can handle. These animal females join this superior male either by choice (lions, gorillas) because they prefer the protection of the strong male against the brutal exposure to isolated males, or are obligated to stick around the superior male for fear of his brutal reactions (baboons). These females are at the disposal of the strong male and have no choice but to submit immediately to any of his sexual requests. Those females who hesitate or oppose the request will be sorry as they may be exposed to the most severe biting or other brutal reactions.

Neck grabbing is common among some animal species such as cats and horses. In fact many animal females (monkeys) have learned to present their rump as a sexual invitation to an angry male in order to quiet him down, and even if the animal male does not respond, this sexual submission indeed satisfies him as it reassures him and confirms his superiority. At the dawn of mankind, the archaic Homo sapiens must not have behaved much differently. Rape rather than courtship, rough sex rather than gentleness, complete disregard for female arousal or, worse, complete ignorance or indifference to it, or even resentment of any female orgasm, and ignoring the presence of the female partner after ejaculation: all these were the rules rather than the exceptions in the life of the cave man. How sparks of mankind penetrated the spirit of primitive Homo sapiens must have extended over millions of years. Depending on the individual, on the culture, and on the time of history, this transformation was complete or incomplete. In some cultures (early North American Indians) rape is tolerated or even glorified. In other cultures it is punishable by death.

One can see that this arrogant male superiority was purely animal in origin and was easily transmitted to primitive man in view of his physical superiority because he was the hunter/provider and was therefore entitled to all kinds of privileges. He was strong, he provided food, and was therefore entitled to all his sexual requests. Somehow late in the prehistory of mankind, it was discovered that ejaculation of the sperm in the vagina led to procreation and that the children also were the father's children. This opened the door for love, intimacy, fidelity, responsibility, formation of the family unit, with emotional feeling replacing or rather coexisting with the brutal animal ancestry. As different family units grouped together to form primitive human society, strict cultural rules became necessary to protect each family unit one from the other, and to prevent any 'superior' male from taking advantage of any other female.

Current sexual behavior can therefore be considered as the combination of three trends.

* First the animal ancestry, in which the biological drives are predominant. It is buried deep within each human male and is active only in dreams and sexual fantasies. In most human males there are only primitive remnants of this animal ancestry. However, it is only skin deep in some men and frequently it resurfaces in terms of rape and other sexual violences.

* Second our cultural background (family, society, law, religion) which imposes strict rules to protect women and the family unit in general. Most human males follow strict rules and have a strict control over their sexual (biological) drives.

* Third there are superior human trends such as emotional feeling, love, respect for another human, which, far beyond social regulations, give a new and elevated aspect to sexuality.

These three trends can exist in different degrees depending on the individual, on the different stages of their life, on the social class, on the culture. One can see that differently from animals human sexuality is very complex in nature.

I am 59 years old, originally from one of the Philippine Islands. I came to the USA at the age of 29 on a student visa. Then I married a Filipino girl here in the USA and I stayed here. On the island where I grew up men were allowed to have more than one wife. My father had four wives. I remember his schedule very well. On Friday morning he got up early for his morning prayer, then we did not see him until four Fridays later. He used to spend one week with each wife on rotation. He had between three to five children with each wife. I barely knew my half-sisters and brothers. My father was wealthy, but he did not work very hard because all he did was collect rent from buildings he owned. He was the absolute master in each house. Our lives were divided into two different parts. The first was the week when he was present. He was generous with each one of us. We all respected him and were scared of him. The house was very silent especially at night when he retired in the bedroom with my mother. Then the house became active again for three weeks in his absence but we had to live in a thrifty way because the amount of money he left my mother for three weeks was variable, depending on his mood and how well his business was going. When he was present nobody was allowed to talk, only to answer when asked a question. He always wanted us around when he was present.

My mother was very respectful and afraid of him. She was supposed to guess whatever he wanted without him asking. Her greatest fear was to have her menstrual period when he was home and her greatest joy was to get pregnant from one of his visits, especially when she gave birth to a boy. I always wondered why she was so scared of him until my sister told me that he had divorced one of his wives (and remarried) because he was displeased with her.

I can tell you I do not get the same treatment from my wife and children. Can you imagine that I take out the garbage everyday, although my wife or my oldest son could do it. Nowadays a man does not get respect from anybody. I love my wife and children but sometimes I feel so angry that I want to take off to my country of birth in the village where I grew up and surround myself with four wives so that I can get the proper respect a man deserves. You know what? Last year a brother of mine from the Philippines came to visit me in the USA. He has only one wife, the second one after he divorced the first one. He could not stand the way my wife and children treated me. He suggested that I return to our village with my family so that my wife and children be reeducated properly. What do you think?

As far as seniors are concerned, the whole concept of male superiority has to be completely reconsidered. Animal remnants are gone, the family unit is terminated, biological determinants have ceased, the senior male is not necessarily the provider anymore nor even necessarily physically stronger. The sexual interrelationship as it exists in animals and even in human adults has completely collapsed. It has to be reconsidered under a completely new basis, mainly the submissive passive woman has disappeared.

Senior Men and Women's Liberation

I am a 70-year old lady. I am having a ball for the last 15-20 years. When I now think of it, my life from 20 to 50 was a nightmare. I got married at the age of 20, and by the age of 30 I had four children. My husband was working hard and was a good provider but sexually speaking he was impossible; all kinds of bizarre sexual requests and sexual positions at any hour of the day and night. He was very fussy about food but, thank God, my mother taught me how to cook. In addition, my mother-in-law developed Alzheimer's disease. My two sisters-in-law and my brothers-in-law did not want to take care of her and my husband said that I was the only one who was good enough to take care of her. Thanks.

Now the air is clear. My mother-in-law passed away and that's good riddance. My husband died of a car accident and may he rest in peace. My youngest child left home to live on her own.

Can you imagine the nerve of my sister-in-law? She has a child with some neurological damage and suggested that I should help her raise him at least on a part-time basis since I am so good with children and since she and her husband have a full time job. I knew too well what giving part-time help meant. It means full-time, the way my siblings-in-law promised help for my mother-in-law and never showed up. I told my sister-in-law in no uncertain terms that I was not a sucker anymore and to go to hell. She was so indignant that she tried to turn all her siblings and even my children against me. That gave me an excellent opportunity to break up with all my in-laws whom I could never stand anyway. Now I am having a good life.

Q: How is your sexual life?

A. Better than ever. No menstruation or fear of pregnancy. No children that may hear. No husband making bizarre requests. I am not promiscuous. I never got involved in a sexual relationship that lasted only one night. My relations with men last on the average of one to two years, with the clear understanding that any one of us is free to go any time we feel like it. I myself broke a few relationships because I lost interest.

Q: What do your children feel about your way of life?

A: The only way not to be criticized by them is to make it clear to them that I am not looking for their approval. My children have no comments although the oldest admires me, and although my youngest daughter, still not married, is somehow critical. I understand her because she barely gets a date.

As can be seen in this case, a senior woman's liberation can take unsuspected turns. She can remain what she was previously or she can take the initiative in the new approach to senior sexuality. Indeed, in senior sexuality many basic elements that determined human sexuality may become obsolete and persist only as a tradition because of fear of change or pure laziness.

For example, the concept of guilt, the fear of satisfying whatever is left of biological trends, may need to be revised, and freedom from previous obligations may be sought. One may be freely attracted in doing what was previously forbidden, because there may be no reasons for this forbidding. One may be free to behave like younger age, or, on the contrary, discover a new aspect of sexuality in old age. As far as senior sexuality is concerned we are in for more surprises, especially on the senior women's sides.

Comparing Adult and Senior Sexuality

It is only after a recapitulation of sexuality in animals and in human adults that we can discuss the sexual changes in senior life (Table 49). Let us first summarize the different aspects of adult human sexuality.

Sex in the adult male is partly biological and partly mental as previously discussed. There is no biological aspect in female sexuality. It is so different from male sexuality that it barely deserves to have the same name. Indeed there are many differences. Male orgasm is 'consecrated' by a biological phenomenon which is ejaculation, while the female orgasm is not 'consecrated' by any biological phenomenon because it is not necessary for procreation.

The male is active and potent in order to perform sex. If he is impotent he cannot have sex. The female, however, can be passive and immobile. There is no such thing as an impotent female. Although modern sexuality has revised this concept by attributing more 'activity' to women, basically impotence is a male attribute.

A woman can perform sexually in a satisfactory manner without displaying much activity if any at all. This is why prostitutes, for instance, can have 10-20 (ore more) sexual acts a day without any effort, while the male has to consecrate each act with an ejaculation and this limits him to only one or a couple of sexual acts a day. On the contrary, male homosexual prostitutes can be penetrated anally many times a day just like a female prostitute. Female passivity in the sexual act is advantageous: a female can easily do without sex unless she feels love for the sexual partner with a desire to please him, feels obligated to accept his sexual requests, or wishes to become pregnant, etc.

Female orgasm is elusive. In summary, a woman can have coitus without orgasm: she is temporarily or permanently frigid.

It is only after getting a broad idea of what sexuality is in adult life that we can approach the meaning of sexuality in senior life. If we could consider that sexual equilibrium is unstable in a separate or combined relationship, then we can understand that this unstable equilibrium will be maintained or become more unstable or fall apart in senior age. On the contrary, the disequilibrium may become more stable in senior age, as each male and/or female senior makes his/her point of view clear.

The man has possibly more time for sex than he had during his adult life when he was working and came home tired and had to get up early to go to work. He does not have to spend the weekend resting, or golfing, or fishing. Now all his time is vacation. He gets up or goes to sleep when he wants and has all the time for any activity of his choice. One therefore would expect an increase in sexual activity in view of the free time, and this is what happens sometimes. Most of the time, however, it remains the same, at least for those people that remain in good health. Others, however, show a decline for all the reasons enumerated. Impotence slowly creeps in: first, erection with limited and/or no ejaculation; partial erection with or without ejaculation; then, complete absence of erection or impotence. During this progressive decline one may or not attempt treatment with Viagra or other herbal medicines. These treatments may work, at least temporarily, or not at all.

As we have discussed, the biological stimuli are almost completely cut off in senior life, and one is left mostly with neurological and cerebral stimuli. Some seniors maintain enough cerebral and neurological stimuli to keep their sexuality going, others do not have the mental capability for it. Let us say that the average male has established a sexual pattern during his adult life and that he has a tendency to maintain it in senior life either by habit, or because he wants to prove to himself or to others that he is still a "man," or because of continuous mental stimulation. These men will maintain or even increase their sexual performance. At the other extreme there may not be enough mental stimuli: one may be inhibited by moral, religious, social, familial, or personal reasons powerful enough to inhibit any cerebral stimuli; and this individual cannot perform sexually, even if there is desire. The retired male (or the male above 55 years of age) is to reevaluate his sex drive in view of major changes in his living conditions.

Changes in senior women are also radical, even more than in men. She no longer procreates, her cycle of her life, which was controlled and regulated by menstrual periods, is over. She has also retired from her work as a mother raising a family, and now she has all the time to reconsider her sexual position.

Often, there may be no change at all. If she was orgasmic, the woman will continue to be, either through heterosexuality, masturbation, or both. If she was not orgasmic or barely orgasmic, she will continue to perform her duties to her husband or her sexual partner. She will keep herself attractive as she has learned during her adult life that sex is much more important to men than women. During her adult life it was more often her husband or sexual partner requesting sex. She knows that sex is necessary to her partner to keep the relationship going.

There may be radical changes however. The woman may give up sex altogether by common agreement with her partner because they both have lost interest in it, or she may never have had an interest in it to begin with. She is now indifferent to sex or it may be painful because her vagina became atretic, and she simply disregards the sexual desire of her partner, submitting to it less and less. This a common source of discord among people of any age, including old age.

The woman may take a liberated attitude, however. The husband is not the boss who determines all sexual behavior. Even if she did not experience orgasm previously, she may want it now. She read in women's magazines that it is the responsibility of the male partner to prepare her properly for orgasm. Many senior women will allow any vaginal penetration only if they had been properly prepared.

In summary, some women keep their same sexual behavior, others give it up, and others feel liberated from any obligation and want to participate in orgasm, or at least have sex their own way.

Birth of Seniors and Sexuality

Currently we are faced with a population that never existed before, at least not to such a large extent, namely the expansion of senior citizens. They extend in number and age and have varying health conditions. Their posture and locomotion may be different, and they eat differently because many have dental problems. They are also faced with incontinence and changes in their sleep patterns. They have minimal, if any, sexual or rather reproductive hormones. They have a different sexuality.

In conclusion, a new race, a new species, the senior Homo sapiens or SHS, is appearing on earth, co-existing with the classic Homo sapiens or HS.

Originally, old age was barely tolerated and seniors depended very much on their children. They were usually neglected and died of malnutrition or disease. But now their number is increasing; they have their own rights, they are protected by the law, they have access to free health care; they have social security and various other benefits derived from their previous job or the wealth they have accumulated. The great evolution of the new millennium is not computers, technology, atomic energy, or space travel, but the appearance and expansion of senior citizenry, and it will determine the future history of mankind. This most significant event in human history started in the western world where people started to live longer and longer, far beyond their reproductive years. This change is spreading all over the world. Seniors are no longer old people waiting to die but "new" people wanting to live or rather wanting to search and define a new way of life adapted to their conditions.

Now we are faced with a new population aging well beyond the usual forties, as previously described. Because seniors are new on earth, their way of life has therefore never been consecrated by nature. Specifically, we do not know about sexuality in old age because there has never been any senior sexuality previously. Senior sexuality cannot be natural because it is new and what is new cannot be natural until it has been consecrated by time, a long time, and after many repetitions, does anything become natural. Until then one can understand the objections coming from everybody, including seniors themselves. Sexually speaking, seniors are faced with many dramatic situations. Almost every senior I discussed sex with always asked me the same questions: "Is it natural for people of my age to have sex?" or "What is the natural way of having sex in people my age?" Another form of the same question is "what kind of sex life do other seniors have?" They apparently want to conform to an existing pattern forgetting that there are none. My answer was always that there is no natural way, and that every senior has to find the solution for himself or herself without referring to any outside authority and without any guilt feelings for practicing (or not practicing) sex this way or that way. This is so because there is nothing outside which to refer. Indeed the factors that determine sexuality in seniors are multiple:

Age
Health (including potency in men, frigidity in women)
Weight (very important for sexual position)
Availability or non-availability of a sex partner
Social and marital status
Guilt feelings about being involved in what they may think they should not do
Mostly, presence or absence of sexual desire
Other factors peculiar to specific individuals

Let us not forget that the two most important factors determining sexual activity in *adult* males and females, namely the presence of sexual hormones (estrogen in females, testosterone in males) and reproductive function, no longer exist in senior citizens.

Senior sexuality has practically nothing to do with sexuality of the preceding years. It has to be discovered, or rather invented, piece by piece. Since seniors are different from each other, one would expect tremendous diversity in their sexual activity, each individual finding what is the most suitable for him/her, but there is no sexual pattern for them to refer to because senior sex never existed previously to any degree to speak of. The question is no longer what is 'normal' but what is the most suitable. Then, what is the most suitable will become 'normal'. There should be what I could call a sexual liberation for senior citizens, free from set patterns usually established by younger generations. Senior sex does not have to copy or be determined by sex of the previous years of adulthood, or by any other authority or person.

Frequency and Diversity of Sex in Seniors

We have seen in our interviews that the most striking characteristic of sexuality in seniors is variation in frequency. Of course, this is also true in the younger generation, but not to such an extent. Sex in young people can more or less be categorized and tabulated as practiced by almost all adult individuals with limited extreme variations. In seniors, it is the opposite. A noticeable segment of seniors have no sex life, but another segment, said to be as large, is sexual with tremendous variations in frequency. I have met men as well as women in their 70s and even into their late 80s, who can challenge the younger generation in their sexual frequency. But, I have also met seniors who have sex only a couple of times a year or not at all. I have met seniors who are promiscuous and who even might be called male or female prostitutes. I have interviewed seniors who are orgasmic to such a frequency that it becomes an embarrassment. Some have reported sexual positions that make the most forward sex videos look amateurish; others are classic in their sexual practice. While some seniors are open about their sexual activity others are prudish, and it takes a lot of patience and skill to get the truth out of them. Such diversity can be explained by the tremendous varying in their health status, but I have also encountered diversity among the healthy as well, although not to such a degree.

Reconsideration of Sexuality in Senior Citizens

During the Middle Ages in Europe and throughout the rest of the world, the average life span was forty, rarely fifty and, as previously shown, life has been expanding ever since. In this study adult life extends from 18 or 20 to 55 years of age, and senior life will start at 55 years of age. In the near future senior life will have a tendency to be equal to adult life. A great mistake is to consider senior life in the light of adult life because they do not have the same mentality, the same emotions, the same interests, etc. Their problems are different, their approach and treatment, if any, are different. Specifically, there is a different sexuality between the two groups. Adult males are sometimes concerned with impotence and adult females with indifference to sex or frigidity. These two problems become minor or may disappear in seniorhood. Some males become concerned about impotence and some females are concerned about frigidity, but not to any extent. On the other extreme, some men, but more so women, have completely lost interest in sex and give it up. Of course, there are all kinds of intermediaries.

Freedom is the ability to consider or reconsider one's behavior or one's mode of action, not necessarily dictated by the established standards such as religion, moral, social, legal and/or familial ones but dictated by new conditions that did not exist previously. This does not mean that one becomes revolutionary. It just means that one is free to reconsider the causes for accepted standards, and not be satisfied anymore when those causes are modified or no longer exist.

Coming to sexual behavior as determined by religious, moral, social, legal and/or familial standards, it is obvious that the reason they existed was to protect the family unit and society in general. Once the core of the family has been terminated and the children are on their own, one is free to revise the existence of the established standards. Even during adult life these sexual standards are nowadays being reconsidered. The application of these sexual standards to seniors has to be reconsidered all the way. There is not much basis for the adult generation to tell seniors: "These are our standards, this is how we behave; therefore, this is how you should behave." Or rather, in terms of sexual behavior, seniors should wonder if they should determine their own standards of behavior or if they should routinely copy the standard of the young generation.

Why Sex in Seniors?

It was, and still is, easy to rule out sexuality for seniors with the classic reasoning that seniors no longer procreate. They are weaker than adults and may not be able to display the necessary physical effort for sexual activity. So, why bother, especially if and when there is no longer a sexual partner (deceased or uncooperative spouse) and one has to get involved in the arduous process of locating a proper sexual partner? Masturbation, homosexuality, prostitutes, affairs, sexual scandals, all place too much stress on seniors as they advance in age and, therefore, could damage their remaining health and expose them to a heart attack or a cerebral hemorrhage. This is how many adults look at senior sexuality, and this is also the prevalent attitude among some seniors themselves who appear to be very confused on the issue. It is in light of the previous study (see Tables 48 and 49) comparing animal versus human sex on one side, and adult versus senior human sexuality on the other, that we can attempt to answer some of these questions.

First, there has never been any criteria for standard or normal senior sexuality to speak of. All one can do, and has been doing, is to ignore or condemn it, speculate, fantasize, or joke about it, or worst of all apply the criteria of adult sexuality to seniors.

Second, we practically have a new species, Senior Homo sapiens (SHS), as opposed to the regular Homo sapiens. We are, therefore, exposed to a tremendous variety of seniors varying in age from 50 to 100, in physical and mental health, and also in sexual desire. Some authors (R. Katzman and J.W. Rowe, Principles of Geriatric Neurology, F.A. Davis Co., Philadelphia, 1992) have wondered why there is such a variety in health conditions among seniors, variety not seen in adults. The answer is simple: natural selection has selected the fittest among adults, but has not, at least not yet, selected the fittest among seniors for survival. I doubt it will ever happen because seniors do not reproduce, and it is through reproduction that natural selection operates.

Third, sexuality and associated love that goes with it are the greatest driving forces that have moved mankind forward. No matter how many problems arise with human sexuality, it is still a fundamental driving force in humans. Therefore, it is completely unjustified to deny sexuality to seniors, thus also denying them any worthwhile activity. No one should stress sexuality to seniors if they are not interested, but neither should anyone deny it to them if they are interested. This is impossible anyway and if one attempts to inhibit it, it becomes hidden, explosive, illegal, predisposed to scandal, and performed anyway. Alcohol prohibition did not work and led to a marked social unrest. Sexual prohibition, even to seniors, would be even worse. One is left in a quandary as to whether there is any role or function left for sexuality in seniors. Everybody has a different opinion including seniors themselves.

The proper attitude is an open mind, open to the tremendous variety of seniors, open to each individual or group that should be free to approach sexuality according to their needs and their wishes. Any other attitude will and does effectively lead to frustration and disappointment.

The mechanical technique of coitus itself is the same as in adulthood. It requires a certain physical effort on the part of seniors, more on the part of the male than the female because the male still has to have an erection, proceed with penetration and successive thrusts and finally ejaculation. The female, although she can be active, can also be completely passive and still have normal sex, just like in adulthood. Here the similarity ends however and the practice of sex in seniors presents tremendous variety.

Sexuality in old age is at a crossroad. It is determined by many factors that are nonexistent in younger people and which currently interfere with it in old age.

It should be emphasized that the reproductive function of sexuality has been rooted in the human mind for thousands of years and is considered by many cultures as the natural and only function of sexuality and any intimate relationship resulting from sex is secondary or even nonexistent, as some religious or philosophical authorities would claim. The question is not crucial in adult life, but becomes crucial with the current wide scale rise of old age and when the reproductive function has completely disappeared. Should seniors, who do not reproduce, practice sex or not, that is the question.

This is the first time that such a separation arises in human history, a time where sexuality has to be looked at as such, completely separate from reproduction. One is left in a quandary when trying to determine the role of sexuality in seniors, and to define the nature of the special relationship created by senior sexuality.

In conclusion, senior sexuality is neither reproductive nor biological. So the function of sex as we age, would leave anyone puzzled and it is no wonder that in old age it is abandoned and condemned by some, hidden by others, and gossiped about by everybody. I repeat, as long as the senior population was not high, the problem was limited to isolated subjects who were dealt with on a case-by-case aspect, mostly by the family. But, the senior population is growing. From being practically nonexistent in the beginning of the 20th century, it now represents 20 percent of the total population and, continuing the current trend, the senior population may equal the adult population by the middle of the present century. By that time there will be as many people practicing sex under the aegis of reproduction and hormones as there will be practicing sex without the aegis of reproduction or hormones!

The very reasons for giving up sex in old age can be the very same reasons to continue or even increase its practice. Indeed, the reproduction function can be a handicap to sexuality. As an obstetrician and gynecologist, I spent more hours teaching my patients about birth control and how to avoid pregnancy rather than how to get pregnant. Pregnancy, menstruation, mood variations during the menstrual cycle, interfere with sexuality. In a family circle, lack of privacy with children around can be a handicap. Tiredness due to an outside job and caring for children can be an obstacle to frequent sexual practice. It is no wonder that some seniors turn to sexuality more frequently than during their adult years.

Senior women who have had limited acquaintance with orgasm during their adult life, will quickly abandon sex during their senior life because they really never had any knowledge of it or any interest in it. Women do not give up sex in senior age, they give up the traditional way of it, i.e. orgasm-less. I rarely met an orgasmic woman who gave up sex in senior age unless she lacked a partner or missed the man she loved so much that she would not consider sex with anyone else.

I insist specifically on female orgasm in senior citizens. I have continuously stressed that female orgasm is a recent and elusive human acquisition. If it had not been there before senior age, it is difficult to bring about, but one should not give up altogether. If it is there at the beginning of senior age, everything should be done to keep it alive, and this includes boyfriends, even paid boyfriends, homosexuality and masturbation. I insist also on the reconsideration of the man's attitude who considers that all he needs is a quick sex act, an ejaculation as soon as possible, and that is the end of it. This male chauvinistic attitude does not work at any age and one better learn to give them up as early as possible in young and adult life. But mostly they do not work in senior age. No permanent male-female relationship will persist under these conditions.

In summary, senior sexuality is a clash against the old way, against the adult generation who has a preconceived idea of what senior sexuality should be. A new thinking, a new approach, based on senior liberation is becoming imperative. It is a senior imperative.

Senior Citizens:
A New Species From The Sexual Point of View

When one analyzes senior sexuality in detail and compares it to adult sexuality, the differences that are found are so enormous that one might rightfully consider that senior sexuality does really belong to a different species. The list of the differences is endless (Tables 48, 49).

The elements of violence and aggressivity so characteristic of animal sexuality and partly still present in adult human sexuality are all gone in senior sexuality. There is no rape, no forced sex, no physical struggle on the part of the senior male trying to impose sex as quickly and as forcefully as possible or on the part of the senior female trying to prevent or delay the sexual act. Courtships are short. The biological struggle imposed by the sexual hormones is all gone. It is now a sexual act under full control of the mind, with complete volition and no forceful decisions. With general weakening in old age, males and females are more or less of similar physical strength and the female can easily protect herself from the forceful male. Specifically on the female side, one no longer sees the many aspects of sexuality seen in the young and adult women. No fear of losing virginity, of being taken advantage of, no fear of pregnancy, or family concerns, no inhibition because of menses, no changes of mood at the time of ovulation or menstruation, no fear of sexually transmitted diseases (rare in seniors) and no fear of unknown sex since they all had previous experiences. The most important aspect of female senior sexuality however is that they have come a long way thinking they are granting men a favor by consenting to sex, although some of them still play "hard-to-get". Since there is really no established pattern of senior sexuality to refer to, for instance there is no book giving instructions, then it should be left to seniors to decide what it should be, without other segments of society making rules for their own convenience and not for the convenience of the seniors. When decisions are made by other than those interested, the door is open to arbitration, prejudice, and stupidity. Problems associated with senior sexuality are there but ignored and hidden.

I always have had difficulty in answering questions and in attempting to relieve seniors' worries. I start with the fact that seniors are new in our generation, at least to such an extent. I stress that it is not the beginning of the end of life, but the beginning of a new segment of life. I show statistically that the senior years are getting longer and longer, and one should not be scared, but should look forward to their future. The way adolescence is a preparation to a meaningful adult life, the same way adult life is a preparation to a meaningful senior life.

I insist that senior life is a new world to be explored, to be discovered like a new continent or a new planet to live on. The conditions of life in this new continent or new planet are new circumstances to be determined by local conditions and not necessarily by the way they lived in the old continent. To put it in simple words, the sexual life of a senior is to be determined by purely personal circumstances such as desire, health, and other circumstances such as finances, and/or the community of seniors he/she lives in.

Mostly, I stress that the sexual life of seniors is not to be a duplicate or an attempted duplicate of what sexual life was in adulthood. The dangers of such a concept is that seniors cannot necessarily duplicate adult life because the living circumstances are different. The other danger of the senior attempting to duplicate the adult sexually, is that the adult becomes immediately the judge of what senior sexual life should be. For instance, adult children become the judge of what the sexual life of their senior parents should or should not be, the same way they try to determine every aspect of their life especially if they live with them. Senior parents should not live with their adult children especially if they plan a sexual life.

If they ask, I try to help seniors explore, discover, even make or invent their own sexual life. I suggest that seniors should discuss their sex life between themselves because they have nothing to learn from sex counselors of the adult group although I know quite a few social workers and even psychologists and psychiatrists who declare themselves specialists in senior sexuality. They should establish their own criteria to practice sex or not. Their sexual life should not adapt to that of adults no more than seniors should determine the adult type. Each senior should determine what fits him or her, disregarding completely what adults do or think seniors should do sexwise. There is no guilt in deviating from anybody else's standard and they should not have any complex feeling of guilt when sexually active in any way.

I insist on the diversity of senior sexual life the same way there is diversity in their life in general. Seniors are very diversified (much more than adults) in terms of their life span, religious background, health, educational background, mental alertness, economical condition, and most of all the availability of a sex partner. This variety will tremendously influence their sexual life. I stress that they are completely free to make their sexual life what they want it to be.

In conclusion, the sexual senior should become practical in terms of who should make sexual advances and propositions, courtship if any, sexual frequency, sexual positions, post-sex behavior, relation of love to sex, relation of companionship to sex, commitment or no commitment, and so on. The list can be extended ad infinitum and the answer to each aspect of senior sexuality is purely personal.

The Union Between Senior Citizens

The partnership between a senior male and female presents characteristics that make this union in a way similar to, in another different from, the union between adults. The union of seniors can be the same one carried from adult age to seniorhood (marriage), or may be a new one established in senior age (remarriage or companionship) (Table 49).

When a couple carry their union from adulthood to seniorhood there is often no change in the relationship. Just as often there is a change in the relationship, or rather there is a showdown and the real relationship surfaces because anything hidden in the previous relationship is now gone since the spouses have retired and all the children have grown up and gone. My opinion has always been that the true relationship in a couple is tested when they are permanently alone, facing each other all day long. This is the real test of a relationship. Those that were intimate and in love become more intimate and more in love. Those that had separate lives and did not know it because they were too busy, now realize they are separate. Those who could not stand each other, now are more separate than ever; some divorce or separate, and some keep up the appearance of living together.

Senior men in general would like to carry their same prior sexual activity, maybe slightly less as they age more. Other senior men who have terminated a previous union (widowhood or separation) either give up sex altogether or try new ventures by looking for a new companion or prostitute in the hope of 'improving' their sex life.

The sexual attitude of senior women is more interesting. It is characterized by two opposite trends. Those women who accepted non-orgasmic sexuality during their adult life had a tendency to liberate themselves by refusing to participate in this non-orgasmic sexuality. Interestingly, now some even want orgasm from their sexual partner by requesting a thorough preparation. We had a group of 29 women who became orgasmic heterosexually for the first time in their life after they reached seniorhood. Some others find and even prefer masturbation rather than (or in addition to) non-orgasmic sexuality. Others finally give up sex altogether to the dismay of their husband or companion, who may either give up sex also, or have an affair. Some women stick to the old pattern just to keep a stable or unstable relationship going, and some still participate in a non-orgasmic sexuality just for the sake of companionship rather than to live alone.

Whatever the attitude of the senior, there is a tendency, or at least an awareness whenever the opportunity arises, of possible liberation from the old pattern of passivity.

Sexuality is the greatest mover of mankind. It is through sexuality that one finds himself or herself, it is through sexuality that one gets the best and the worst out of himself or herself. Most of all it is through sexuality that we learn to relate or not to each other, to love or hate each other. This is well known to be true in adolescence and adulthood, and now that all of us are moving at one time or another into seniorhood this also remains true in senior age. The discovery of oneself and others is just as real in senior age the way it was in previous age. Even if sexuality is performed to a lesser degree or given up in old age, the values acquired in earlier age still persist for better or worse.

The gentleman who as an adult always treasured and cared for his female partner, who approached her gently and delicately always aware of her shyness and her desires, and who through his skill and patience managed to lead her to a sexual climax whenever she desired it, will remain the same as a senior and his companionship will always be sought. This senior will be quickly forgiven for increasingly limited sexual performance.

Reversely, the gentlemen who as an adult was selfish and self-centered, who approached the female body only as an object for sexual stimulation, got drunk before sex to bring a truncated ego to the sexual act, turned his back immediately after ejaculation, and kept going from one sexual affair to another with the elusive hope of finding the perfect match, will remain the same in senior age regardless of his sexual achievements or lack of. He could use Viagra, baculum, and other gadgets or other herbs and medications, but all he will do is increase his frustration and that of his sexual partners. This senior gentleman may be sought for his money or social position, his hollow companionship, or other egotistic and superficial reasons, and he may live in an illusionary world of sexual success. Yet, I do not mean that there is no real indications for Viagra, baculuum, and all the other gadgets and herbs.

We can make similar general remarks about senior women. Women in adolescence and adult life started sexuality with hope, apprehension, illusion and with the feeling that they were holding within them some powerful treasure. Some women will fulfill their aspirations in general, and their sexual life in particular. They manage, after careful search, to find the perfect man with whom they will explore and discover the world of heterosexuality and heterosexual orgasm. They learn to give without pushing, and receive without taking. It is unbelievable how these exceptional women are intuitively perceived and selected regardless of age and beauty. A potentially orgasmic woman will always find how to achieve orgasm.

Some other women will never achieve climax although they may be under the illusion of having orgasm or multiple orgasms. They may be more preoccupied with the impression that they hold the power of controlling male sexuality rather than building their own climax, which may be slow to come and needs to be progressively built over time. They may just play being attractive or be more concerned about being seductive. Their way of life is in the direction of clothing, jewelry, shoes, hairstyles, manicures, pedicures, tone of voice, artificial or natural smile, and so on. They may be satisfied with being irresistible. They just want to be loved and constantly ask for it without return. They may simulate orgasm in order to build the male ego and hide their own frustrations. They do not have the courage to progressively build love, and are afraid to love and to be loved.

The reason we expanded on the above description is because whatever a person is in adult life, he/she will tend to remain so in senior life. Good or bad habits, sexual or otherwise, are carried over into senior stage. In fact, they often become reinforced because seniors have all the time in the world to express their deep personality as they are free from multiple obligations that plagued adult life. When they reach senior age, seniors have the opportunity to realize or not all the plans and dreams they made during adulthood but did not have the opportunity to execute. Some may have planned to give up sex, but others may have planned to go on a sexual rampage. Therefore, the best and the worst may surface in senior age. Of course, this is only an opportunity in senior age and many, if not most, miss it.

This does not mean at all that we are stuck in senior age with the concepts we acquired during our adolescent and adult life. On the contrary, seniorhood is a new opportunity to reconsider and reevaluate all the values of life including the sexual values. One may choose to give up some values including sex, to keep other values including sex, or may totally reconsider any value including sex under a new light and adapted to a new age without any obligation to stick to previously established concepts.

Women specifically are vulnerable in terms of orgasmic sexuality, much more than men. The male orgasm is practically natural because it is built into the reproductive organs and culminates in ejaculation so that one can say that male orgasm is physiological. But female orgasm is not built on any organ and does not fulfill any physiological function. It has to be built de novo early in sexual life or may never be built. If not present, this will not interfere with her sexual and reproductive life. However, when a woman of any age meets the proper sex partner there is a great chance for orgasm to appear. A few will discover climax only in senior life, others may discover climax in senior age (or before) through masturbation.

Final Impression

Should the sex life in seniors (or at any age for that matter) be controlled by religion, ethical, moral, social or familial considerations, or should it be more individualized and liberal as long as it is between two consenting individuals of different or same sex? Let us consider once more how adult sex is different from senior sex. What I call "free sex" always had to be controlled in adult life for many reasons, the most important being fear of pregnancy and fear of venereal diseases. But now with the advent of birth control, pregnancy can be controlled and avoided if so desired. With the discovery of antibiotics, syphilis, which used to be a lifetime disease, is now cured with one single penicillin injection. All other sexually transmitted diseases (including HIV) can be treated and/or avoided with proper precautions. The sexual taboos, which were inherited from previous generations have, therefore, to be revised even for the adult group. The adult generation has freed itself already from these taboos and it is completely unrealistic to apply them to seniors.

To some degree, society was right to control sexual activity in order to protect the family unit (spouse and children) and to prevent the strongest man from taking over any woman he sexually desired, the way it occurs in animals. If strong men had this freedom, society would fall apart. But seniors (men as well as women) barely need any of these protections, and the social taboos concerning sexuality do not necessarily apply to them and should be reconsidered as far as they are concerned.

I have no explanation as to why sexuality in seniors is frowned upon almost by everyone and considered ridiculous, outrageous, and out of place. If seniors are not genuinely interested in sex, so be it. But, if they are interested in it, and in view of their increasing numbers, any attempt to inhibit it leads to concealed practices such as affairs, secret liaisons, visits to prostitutes, and sexual scandals, to name only a few. A more open attitude is healthier and to everyone's advantage.

Sexual problems in seniors are therefore not to be ignored because they appear to be more numerous and more complex. True, with declining health, increasing impotence, and lack of sexual interest, seniors are at a sexual disadvantage. But increased free time, possibility to give more attention to their health, increased experience, different sexual postures, promise of more and better sexual stimulants, seniors are not so much at a disadvantage, especially for the men who, after all, have more opportunity to meet the proper sexual mate than at any other time in their prior life.

Seniors are therefore at a crossroad, sexually speaking. They can walk away from sex, they can keep doing or trying to do what they did before being seniors, or they can take a fresh and novel look at sexuality. After all, they are aware how the younger generation is confused and mixed up about sexuality. They do not have to inherit this disorganization. On the contrary, they are in a position to deal with the numerous problems facing human sexuality. At least they are in a position to do so. Their sexuality does not have the same bindings and the same obligations of a younger age. Therefore we end up with this strange conclusion, as bizarre as it seems: seniors can go forward, can be the leaders in the new sexual revolution, taking advantage, I repeat, of their free time, their experience, improved health and even the use of sexual stimulants. Samantha from *Sex and the City* does not have to turn her back to the senior man in terms of sexuality. She can look forward in that sexual relation to learn more about sex. *Sex and the City* will become "Sex in the Senior

Community." Indeed, we have demonstrated all along during this study how female orgasm is elusive, difficult to reach, hard and capricious to elicit. Orgasmic sexuality in the female is an unresolved problem from the evolutionary point of view, and generations of all ages are struggling with it. In a more limited way, there is a similar problem in male orgasm. We now have a new generation, I will not hesitate to call it a new species that has been added to the currently existing human species. I mean Senior Homo sapiens or SHS. This new species has to tackle all human problems, and they already demonstrated their capability and even superiority in this matter. There is no reason why they should not and there are many reasons why they should also approach the problem of human sexuality.

TABLES

Table 1
Distribution Population (in millions) 1996 - U.S.A.

Age	Male	Female	Total
0-4	12.3	12.7	25
5-9	10	9.6	19.6
10-14	9.8	9.2	19
15-19	9.6	9.1	18.7
20-24	9.0	8.3	17.3
25-29	9.6	9.5	19.1
30-34	10.7	10.8	21.5
35-39	11.2	11.4	22.6
40-44	10.2	10.4	20.6
45-49	9.0	9.4	18.4
50-54	7.8	8.2	16
55-59	5.4	5.9	11.3
60-64	4.7	5.3	10
65-69	4.4	5.2	9.6
70-74	3.8	5.0	8.8
75-79	3.0	3.9	6.9
80-84	1.5	3.1	4.6
85+	1.2	2.4	3.6
Total	133.2	139.4	272.6

Summary of Senior U.S. Population 272.6 (in millions) in 1996

Young	= 82.3	30.2%
Adult	= 135.5	49.7%
55 yrs old and above	= 54.8	20.1%

Of senior population in millions: (55+):
24.0 (males) 43.8%
30.8 (females) 56.2%

Ratio senior male/senior female 24/30.8 = 77.9%

Table 2
Life Expectancy (Average Life Span) - U.S.A.

	Female	Male
1902	48	46
1930	59	56
1969	74	67
1996	79	73
2002	80	77

Table 3

Distribution by Age of the Senior Population Approached for this Study

Ages	Total	55-59	60-64	65-69	70-74	75-79	80-84	85+
Repartition by age	3396	730	672	588	537	428	251	190
% of seniors by age	100%	21.5%	19.8%	17.3%	15.8%	12.6%	7.4%	5.6%
Male	1526	352	287	294	227	203	96	69
%	100%	23.1%	18.8%	19.3%	14.9%	13.3%	6.2%	4.5%
Female	1870	378	385	294	310	225	157	121
%	100%	20.2%	20.6%	15.7%	16.6%	12.0%	8.4%	6.5%

N.B. The approached population (3396 seniors) is composed of:
1526 senior males or 44.9%
1870 senior females or 55.1%

Table 4
Distribution by Age of U.S. Senior Population in 1996
(figures in millions)

Ages	Total	55-59	60-64	65-69	70-74	75-79	80-84	85+
Repartition by age	54.8	11.3	10	9.6	8.8	6.9	4.6	3.6
% of seniors by age	100%	20.6%	18.2%	17.5%	16.1%	12.6%	8.4%	6.6%
Male	24	5.4	4.7	4.4	3.8	3.0	1.5	1.2
%	100%	22.5%	19.6%	18.3%	15.8%	12.5%	6.3%	5.0%
Female	30.8	5.9	5.3	5.2	5.0	3.9	3.1	2.4
%	100%	19.5%	17.2%	16.9%	16.2%	12.7%	10.1%	7.7%

N.B. U.S. population 55 yrs old +, in 1996 was 24.0 million males
30.8 million females
54.8 total

or it was 24.0 / 54.8 = 43.8% males
30.8 / 54.8 = 56.2% females

Table 5
Senior Subject Eligible and Not Eligible for the Study

Total representative population, 3396: 1526 males; 1870 females

A. Eligible for study			
Accepted interview on first approach	1186		
Accepted interview on subsequent approach	1006		
Completed questionnaire only (anonymous)	387		
Satisfactory telephone interview	143		
Total population eligible for study	2722	2722	(80.2%)
B. Not Eligible for study			
Refused interview or limited interview	267		(7.8%)
Mental handicap: (senility, paranoia) (early dementia) (early Alzheimer)	200		(5.9%)
Physical handicap	207		(6.1%)
Total not eligible for study	674	674	(19.8%)
Grand total		3396	(100%)

Table 6
Repartition by Race

	Male		Female		Total	
Total approached population	1526	100%	1870	100%	3396	100%
White	1262	82.7%	1537	82.2%	2798	82.4%
Afro-American	118	7.7%	174	9.3%	292	8.6%
Other	146	9.6%	159	8.5%	306	9.0%

Table 7
Religious Background

Total investigated population	3396	100%
Protestant	2377	70%
Catholic	350	10.3%
Jewish	306	9.0%
Others	68	2.0%
No Affiliation	295	8.7%

Table 8
Origin of the Different Subjects

Community living institution (9)	
Gated community	913
Room and board	438
Assisted living	225
Nursing home	122
Total	1748
Private practice (4)	863
Clinic OPD Centers (3)	785
Gynecological clinic	
Urology clinic	
General medicine	
Total	3396

Table 9
Mode of Living

	Male	Female	Total
Living in a private apartment or home:			
Married	267	252	619
Living with companion or 'steady' dating	109	113	122
Living with family (sibling, children)	193	207	400
Living with others	106	147	253
Living alone	150	181	331
Living in a retirement community such as gated community, retirement community, room and board community, preassisted living, assisted living, nursing home:			
Married	238	258	596
Living with partner or 'steady' dating	110	99	109
Living with family (sibling, children)	62	105	167
Living with others	85	148	233
Living alone	206	360	566
Total	1526	1870	3396
Percentage	44.9%	55.1%	100%

Table 10
Distribution by Age of Interviewed Population

Ages	Total	55-59	60-64	65-69	70-74	75-79	80-84	85+
Repartition by age	2722	655	589	489	438	332	150	69
% of seniors by age	100%	24.1%	21.6%	17.3%	16.1%	12.2%	5.5%	2.5%
Male	1239	315	275	231	203	144	53	18
%	100%	25.4%	22.2%	18.6%	16.4%	11.6%	4.3%	1.5%
Female	1483	340	314	258	235	188	97	51
%	100%	22.9%	21.2%	17.4%	15.8%	12.8%	6.5%	3.4%

Table 11
Attitude of Young and Adults Concerning their Sexuality
When They Will Reach Senior Age

	Male	(%)	Female	(%)	Total	(%)
Total people approached	569		933		1502	
Refused interview or unsatisfactory interview	165	(29.0%)	284	(30.4%)	449	(30.0%)
Total satisfactorily interviewed	404	(71.0%)	649	(69.6%)	1053	(70.0%)
Will abstain (religious, social, familial, personal reasons)	86	(21.3%)	250	(38.5%)	336	(31.9%)
Same, but fearful of being impotent (male) or frigid (female)	178	(44.1%)	123	(19.0%)	301	(28.6%)
Same, but fearful of not satisfying partner	121	(30%)	108	(16.6%)	229	(21.7%)
Will indulge more because of less inhibition (menses, pregnancy, privacy, job)	77	(19.1%)	104	(16.0%)	181	(17.2%)
Do not know	65	(16.1%)	105	(16.2%)	170	(16.1%)
Total number of answers	527	(130%)	690	(106%)	1217	(112%)

N.B. Some subjects gave more than one answer

Table 12

Attitude of Young and Adult Towards Sexuality of their Senior Relatives

	Male	(%)	Female	(%)	Total	(%)
Total people approached	569		933		1502	
Refused interview or unsatisfactory interview	186	(32.7%)	255	(27.3%)	441	(29.4%)
Total satisfactorily interviewed	383	(67.3%)	678	(72.7%)	1061	(70.6%)
1. Should abstain completely	154	(40.2%)	407	(60.0%)	561	(52.9%)
2. Restrain and be discrete about it	59	(15.4%)	205	(30.3%)	264	(24.9%)
3. Same as adult	116	(30.3%)	154	(22.7%)	270	(25.5%)
4. More than adults because freer	46	(12.0%)	52	(7.7%)	98	(9.2%)
5. It is up to them	144	(37.6%)	168	(24.8%)	312	(29.4%)
6. Embarrassed in discussing the subject	107	(28.0%)	271	(40.0%)	378	(35.6%)
7. Do not know	69	(18.0%)	135	(20.0%)	204	(19.2%)
8. Total number of answers	695	(181%)	1392	(205%)	2087	(197%)

N.B. Some subjects gave more than one answer

Table 13

Children's Knowledge of their Senior Parents Sexual Activity

	Sons	(%)	Daughters	(%)	Total	(%)
Total son/daughter approached	340		625		965	
Refused interview or unsatisfactory interview	38	(11.2%)	57	(9.1%)	95	(9.8%)
Total interviewed	302	(88.8%)	568	(90.9%)	870	(90.2%)
Seniors are sexually active	58	(19.2%)	41	(7.2%)	99	(11.4%)
Suspect seniors are sexually active	41	(13.6%)	52	(9.2%)	93	(10.7%)
Doubt seniors are sexually active	32	(10.6%)	67	(11.8%)	99	(11.4%)
Seniors are not sexually active	59	(19.5%)	218	(38.4%)	277	(31.8%)
Do not know	112	(37.1%)	190	(33.5%)	302	(34.7%)

Table 14

To the Senior's Knowledge, is their Sexual Activity Known to their Children

	Male (%)		Female (%)		Total (%)	
Total senior sexually active	931		471		1402	
Children know parents sexually active	255	(27.4%)	49	(10.4%)	304	(21.7%)
Children suspect parents sexually active	178	(19.1%)	70	(14.9%)	248	(17.7%)
Children doubt parents sexually active	62	(6.7%)	28	(5.9%)	90	(6.4%)
Children are convinced their parents are sexually inactive	317	(34.0%)	227	(48.2%)	544	(38.8%)
Parents do not know if children are aware or not	119	(12.8%)	97	(20.6%)	216	(15.4%)

Table 15
To the Senior's Knowledge, is their Sexual Inactivity Known to their Children

	Men (%)		Women (%)		Total (%)	
Total senior sexually inactive	257		836		1093	
Children know parents sexually inactive	208	(80.9%)	740	(88.5%)	948	(86.7%)
Children suspect parents sexually inactive	0	(0%)	10	(1.2%)	10	(0.9%)
Children doubt parents sexually inactive	14	(5.5%)	0	(0%)	14	(1.3%)
Children are convinced their parents are sexually inactive	27	(10.5%)	39	(4.7%)	66	(6.0%)
Parents do not know if children are aware of their sexual inactivity	8	(3.1%)	47	(5.6%)	55	(5.0%)

Table 16

Concern of Seniors About Outside Opinion Regarding their Sexual Activity **

	Male (%)	Female (%)	Total (%)
Total interviewed	1239	1483	2722
1. Should abstain completely (religious, social, family reasons)	232 (18.7%)	593 (40.0%)	825 (30.3%)
2. Should restrain and be very discrete about it	118 (9.5%)	291 (19.6%)	409 (15.0%)
3. Should have as much sexual activity as before age 55	608 (49.1%)	310 (20.9%)	918 (33.7%)
4. Should have more sexual activity	24 (2.0%)	74 (5.0%)	99 (3.6%)
5. Senior should make own decision	587 (47.4%)	294 (19.8%)	881 (32.4%)
6. Embarrassed in discussing the subject	15 (1.2%)	265 (17.9%)	280 (10.3%)
7. Do not know	193 (15.6%)	286 (19.3%)	479 (17.6%)
8. Total number of answers	1778 (144%)	2113 (143%)	3891 (143%)

** Some subjects gave more than one answer

Table 17
Sexual Profile of the Senior Population

	Male (N=1239)		Female (N=1483)		Total (N=2722)	
Heterosexual:	931	(75.1%)	471	(31.8%)	1402	(51.5%)
Orgasmic	721	(58.3%)	190	(12.8%)	911	(33.5%)
Poorly or non-orgasmic	210	(16.9%)	281	(19.0%)	491	(18.0%)
Homosexual	3	(0.3%)	0		3	(0.2%)
Masturbation	48	(3.9%)	176	(11.9%)	224	(8.2%)
No sexual activity	257	(20.7%)	836	(56.3%)	1093	(40.1%)

Table 18
Variation of Senior Sexuality by Age (Heterosexuality Only)

A. Male (see also figure 3)

	Total	55-59	60-64	65-69	70-74	75-79	80-84	85+
Repartition by age (a)	1236	312	275	231	203	144	53	18
Active hetero-sexual (b)	931	278	239	175	133	74	25	7
Percentage sexually active b:a	75.3%	89.1%	86.9%	75.8%	65.5%	51.4%	47.2%	38.9%

B. Female (see also Figure 3)

	Total	55-59	60-64	65-69	70-74	75-79	80-84	85+
Repartition by age (a)	1483	340	309	258	240	178	107	51
Active hetero-sexual (b)	471	114	96	105	68	49	28	11
Percentage heterosexual (b:a)	31.8%	33.5%	31.1%	40.7%	8.3%	27.5%	26.2%	21.2%

Table 19
Percentage sexual activity at different ages (N = 1236)
(3 homosexuals not included)

Age distribution	Total	55-59	60-64	65-69	70-74	75-79	80-84	85 +
Male population (N = 1236, 3 homosexuals not included)								
Total nbr by age (a)	1236 (100%)	312 (25.2%)	275 (22.2%)	231 (8.7%)	203 (16.4%)	144 (11.7%)	53 (4.3%)	18 (1.5%)
Nbr hetero-orgasmic (b)	721 (58.3%)	240 (76.9%)	203 (73.8%)	161 (69.7%)	57 (28.1%)	33 (22.9%)	21 (39.6%)	6 (33.3%)
Nbr mastur-bation (c)	48 (3.9%)	15 (4.8%)	8 (2.9%)	11 (4.8%)	7 (3.4%)	4 (2.8%)	2 (3.8%)	1 (5.6%)
Nbr poor or no orgasm (d)	210 (17.0%)	38 (12.2%)	36 (13.1%)	14 (6.1%)	76 (37.4%)	41 (28.5%)	4 (7.6%)	1 (5.6%)
Nbr no sexuality (a)	257 (20.8%)	19 (6.1%)	28 (10.2%)	45 (19.5%)	63 (31.0%)	66 (45.8%)	26 (49.1%)	10 (55.6%)
Female population (N = 1483)								
Total distri-bution by age (a)	1483 (100%)	340 (22.9%)	314 (22.2%)	258 (17.4%)	235 (15.8%)	188 (12.7%)	97 (6.5%)	51 (3.4%)
Nbr hetero orgasmic (b)	190 (12.8%)	35 (10.3%)	36 (11.5%)	37 (14.3%)	28 (11.9%)	35 (18.6%)	11 (11.3%)	8 (15.7%)
Nbr mastur-bation (c)	176 (11.9%)	34 (7.1%)	14 (8.6%)	19 (11.2%)	36 (15.3%)	46 (21.3%)	13 (13.4%)	14 (13.7%)
Nbr non-orgasmic (d)	281 (18.9%)	79 (26.2%)	50 (15.0%)	68 (22.5%)	40 (17.0%)	14 (10.6%)	17 (17.5%)	3 (19.6%)
Nbr no sexuality (e)	836 (56.4%)	192 (56.5%)	204 (65.0%)	134 (51.9%)	131 (55.7%)	93 (49.5%)	56 (57.7%)	26 (51.0%)

Table 20
Weekly Frequency of Coitus Among Sexually Active Seniors

I. Male

	Total	55-59	60-64	65-69	70-74	75-79	80-84	85+
a) Repartition by age of sexually active	931	278	239	175	133	74	25	7
Average	2.4	3.2	2.2	2.5	2.1	1.2	0.5	0.3
Range	7-0.1	6-1	7-1	7-0.5	4-0.3	4-0.1	3-0.2	2-0.1
b) Orgasmic	721	240	203	161	57	33	21	6
Average	2.9	3.9	2.6	2.4	2.2	1.3	0.8	0.6
Range	70.4	7-2	7-2	7-1	4-1.2	4-0.5	3-0.5	2-0.4
c) Poorly orgasmic	210	38	36	14	76	41	4	1
Average	0.7	1.0	0.8	0.7	1.1	0.6	0.1	0.1
Range	2-0.1	1.4-0.3	1.6-0.3	1-0.5	1.4-0.7	0.8-0.4	0.1	0.1

II. Female

	Total	55-59	60-64	65-69	70-74	75-79	80-84	85+
a) Repartition by age	471	114	96	105	68	49	28	11
Average	1.6	1.9	1.8	1.6	1.2	1.2	0.8	0.6
Range	5-0.1	5-0.5	4-0.2	3-0.5	4-0.7	3-0.7	3-0.1	2-0.1
b) Orgasmic	190	35	36	37	28	35	11	8
Average	1.8	2.3	1.9	1.8	2.0	1.5	1.7	0.8
Range	5-0.8	5-1	4-0.4	5-1.5	4-1	3-0.7	3-0.4	2-0.7
c) Non-orgasmic	281	79	60	68	40	14	17	3
Average	0.8	1.7	1.7	1.0	0.7	0.4	0.2	0.1
Range	1-0.1	3-0.2	3-0.2	3-0.2	2-0.1	2-0.1	1-0.1	1-0.1

Table 21
Comparing Sexual Activity Before and After Age 55

	A. Male			B. Female		
	Before 55	After 55	Variations	Before 55	After 55	Variations
Total population	1239	1239		1483	1483	
Heterosexual	1041	931	-10.6%	1050	471	-55%
a) orgasmic	924	721	-22%	238	190	-20.2%
b) non-orgasmic	117	210	+80%	812	281	-65.4%
Homosexual	9	3	-66.7%	4	0	-100%
Masturbation	57 (4.6%)	48 (3.9%)	-15.8%	70 (4.7%)	176 (11.9%)	+151%
No interest	114	180	+58%	143	330	+132%
No partner	18	77	+328%	216	506	+134%

Table 22
Heterosexual Positions in Different Ages and Percentage of Frequency

A. Male

Age distribution	Adult	55-59	60-64	65-69	70-74	75-79	80-84	85+
Nbr male heterosexual	826	278	239	175	133	74	25	7
Sexual position 1	736 (89%)	175 (63%)	178 (74%)	98 (56%)	31 (23%)	15 (20%)	6 (24%)	2 (29%)
Sexual position 2	215 (26%)	78 (28%)	53 (22%)	57 (33%)	29 (22%)	9 (12%)	5 (20%)	1 (14%)
Sexual position 3	179 (22%)	74 (27%)	10 (4%)	2 (1%)	0 (0%)	0 (0%)	0 (0%)	0 (0%)
Sexual position 4	109 (13%)	60 (22%)	97 (41%)	26 (15%)	25 (19%)	14 (19%)	2 (8%)	1 (14%)
Sexual position 5	197 (28%)	111 (40%)	130 (54%)	76 (43%)	60 (45%)	36 (49%)	14 (56%)	3 (43%)
Sexual position 6	426 (52%)	37 (13%)	42 (18%)	20 (11%)	12 (9%)	4 (5%)	1 (4%)	0 (0%)
B. Female								
Nbr female heterosexual	425	124	83	95	68	55	28	18
Sexual position 1	320 (75%)	87 (70%)	35 (42%)	48 (51%)	25 (51%)	22 (50%)	12 (40%)	6 (33%)
Sexual position 2	215 (51%)	42 (34%)	18 (22%)	14 (15%)	14 (21%)	10 (18%)	5 (18%)	3 (17%)
Sexual position 3	198 (47%)	23 (19%)	5 (6%)	0 (0%)	0 (0%)	0 (0%)	0 (0%)	0 (0%)
Sexual position 4	43 (10%)	38 (31%)	13 (17%)	9 (9%)	7 (10%)	3 (5%)	0 (0%)	1 (6%)
Sexual position 5	100 (24%)	52 (42%)	35 (42%)	37 (39%)	32 (47%)	22 (40%)	11 (39%)	8 (44%)
Sexual position 6	207 (49%)	34 (27%)	17 (20%)	8 (8%)	8 (12%)	1 (2%)	0 (0%)	0 (0%)

Table 23
After Sex Behavior (Heterosexual Only) *

A. Men

	Before Age 55		After Age 55	
Interviewed population	396	%	931	%
Wanted prolonged coitus	332	83.8	366	39.3
Waits for partner to reach orgasm	212	53.5	212	22.8
Wants to be alone (turns back, falls asleep)	131	33.1	213	22.9
Wants to leave, walk away	106	26.8	117	12.6
Keeps talking casually	61	15.9	388	41.7
Keeps hugging	37	9.3	47	5.0
Feeling of ecstasy	10	2.5	98	10.5
Their sexual life affects general life	365	92.2	213	22.9
Ambiguous answer or do not know	76	19.2	75	8.1

B. Women

	Before Age 55		After Age 55	
Interviewed population	513	%	471	%
Want to extend coitus beyond ejaculation in order to reach orgasm	374	72.9	191	40.6
Very frustrated when unable to reach climax, tendency to blame partner	308	60.0	122	25.9
Do not search for climax, are casual about coitus	62	12.1	189	40.1
Definitely want to extend romance beyond coitus (hugging, kissing)	332	64.7	57	12.1
Annoyed with coitus and relieved when over	27	5.3	103	21.9
Feeling of ecstasy even when no climax	40	7.8	47	10.0
Their sexual life affects their general life	417	81.3	170	36.1
Ambiguous answers and do not know	115	22.4	28	5.9

* Many gave more than one answer

Table 24
Sexual Activity (of lack of it) Within Marriage

	Husbands	Wives
Sexual activity only with spouse	125	125
Outside regular affair	30	11
Female or male prostitute	40	3
Masturbation	13	40
Homosexuality	2	0
Interested, but inactive spouse, no outside partner	15	41
No interest in sex	25	30
Total	250	250

Table 25
Concern About Physical Appearance *

A. Male

Total interviewed	1239	%
Using surgery to appear young:		
plastic surgery	11	0.9
hair transplant	7	0.6
genital surgery such as baculum or penis elongation	14	1.1
Viagra and/or other stimulating medication	218	17.6
Excessive attention to clothing, shaving, hair style	73	5.9
Excessive concern about looking old	115	9.3
Lying about age	206	16.6
Never telling age	277	22.4

B. Female

Total interviewed	1483	
Using surgery to appear young:		
plastic surgery once	112	7.5
plastic surgery more than once	45	3.0
plastic surgery for tighter vagina (vaginal plastic)	76	5.2
Viagra or other stimulating medication	129	8.7
Excessive attention to clothing, hair style, make-up	578	39.0
Excessive concern about looking old	733	49.4
Lying about age	437	29.5
Never telling age	1186	80

* Some give more than one answer

Table 26
Use of Viagra and the Like in Seniors

	Senior Men		Senior Women		Total	
Total population	1239		1483		2722	
Total senior users	218	(100%)	129	(100%)	347	(100%)
Great success	75	(34.4%)	23	(17.8%)	98	(28.2%)
Limited success	61	(28.0%)	25	(19.4%)	86	(24.8%)
No success	82	(37.6%)	81	(62.8%)	163	(47.0%)

Table 27
Health Concerns Associated with Sexual Activity in Seniors *

	Male	Female	Total
Total interviewed	1239	1483	2722
Obesity	210	317	527
Diabetes	186	225	411
Hypertension	173	161	334
Cardiac condition	64	124	188
Arthritis	410	404	814
Prostate (male)/genital prolapse (female)	183	75	264
Mental illness	21	43	64
Taking different medications	436	513	949
Weakness	192	316	508
Apathy	210	406	616
Total complaints	1655	2071	3726
Number of complaints per senior	1.33	1.40	1.37

* Many seniors have more than one health concerns
* This table does not include the seriously ill seniors (see Table 5) who are not included in this study.

Table 28

Health and Senior Sexuality (All Types of Sexuality Included)

	Senior Male	Sexually Active		Senior Female	Sexually Active	
Total senior population	1239	983	(79.3%)	1483	647	(43.6%)
Seniors with health concerns (a)	670	503	(75.1%)	656	281	(42.8%)
Senior without health concerns (b)	569	479	(84.2%)	827	366	(44.3%)
Difference (b-a)			9.1%			1.5%

Table 29
Duration of Sexual Abstention Among Sexually Active Seniors

	Male	%	Female	%
Interviewed senior population	931		471	
Did abstain up to 1 month only	93	10	6	1.3
Did abstain up to 3 months only	407	24.8	67	14.2
Did abstain up to 6 months only	231	43.7	89	18.9
Did abstain up to 1 year only	114	12.2	184	39.1
Did abstain for more than 1 year	86	9.2	125	26.5

Table 30
Senior Male Evaluation of Coitus

Total heterosexual senior population	931	%
Limited to one female partner	803	86.3
Will approach only consenting female partner	707	75.9
General body touching by female partner	334	35.9
Hand penis (hetero-masturbation)	585	59.6
Mouth-penis	108	11.6
Sexual play only (occasionally satisfied with)	73	7.8
Short duration of penetration	101	10.8
Incomplete erection	202	21.7
Difficult or no ejaculation	210	22.6
Satisfactory duration of penetration	612	65.7
Indifferent to sex (only to satisfy partner)	94	10.1
Generally satisfied with sex	787	84.5
Looks forward to mutual orgasm	506	54.3
Generally frustrated	180	19.3

* Many subjects gave multiple reasons

Table 31
Senior Female Evaluation of Coitus *

Total heterosexual senior population	471	%
Limited to one male partner	452	96
Consent to sex only when in the mood	207	44
General good preparation by male partner	230	49
Touching of body, of breasts, by partner	268	56.9
Finger/vagina (hetero-masturbation)	205	43.5
Mouth/vagina	133	28.3
Occasionally satisfied with sex play only	104	22.1
Sexual act is too short	166	35.2
Satisfactory duration of penetration	309	65.6
Frequent culmination to orgasm	190	40.3
Infrequent or no orgasm	281	59.7
Indifferent to sex (only to satisfy partner)	135	28.7
Annoyed with sex, avoids it as much as possible	150	31.8
Painful act	62	13.2
Masturbates before and/or after coitus to reach orgasm	198	42.0
Generally satisfied with sex	308	65.6
Looks forward to mutual orgasm	302	64.2
Generally frustrated	142	29.7

* Many subjects gave multiple reasons

Table 32
Motivation for Heterosexual Activity *

	Male	%	Female	%
Total heterosexual senior population	931		471	
Biological urge	685	73.6%	172	36.5%
Need to feel young	379	40.7%	130	27.6%
Habit carried from previous age	266	28.6%	230	48.8%
Need to satisfy partner	88	9.5%	172	36.6%
Associated with love	203	21.8%	311	66%
Other reasons	70	7.5%	77	16.3%
Do not know	19	2%	3	0.6%

* 1) Masturbation and homosexuality are not included
2) Many subjects give multiple reasons (average of two reasons per subject)

Note: "Hunting" of woman by man in senior age is nothing but carried from adult age. Women looking after man is not uncommonly sexual but also looking for other goals: companionship, support, high status, combination.

Table 33
Reasons for Sexual Inactivity **

	Male	Female
Total population	1239	1483
No sexuality	257	836
Percentage no sexuality	20.7%	56.3%
Hesitant in approaching	7	18
Hesitant in being approached	16	33
Looking for but does not find partner	15	393
Looking mostly for companion, no sex	4	386
Wants to be supported	3	254
Looking for social status of a companion	35	166
Religious objections	7	46
Moral objections	2	46
Family objections	0	257
No interest in sex	38	182
Interest in sex but painful	0	45
Hostile to sex	0	31
Interest but impotence/frigidity	71	182
Does not want to get involved	33	20
Had previous bad experience	20	67
Fear of not being able to perform	31	8
Prefer to be alone	33	103
Too old looking to be sexually attractive	6	198
Physically unable to perform	39	15
Do not know	22	160
	379	2610

** Many gave more than one answer

Table 34
Disequilibrium in Male/Female Senior Population

	Total	55-59	60-64	65-69	70-74	75-79	80-84	85+
Repartition by age	2722	655	589	489	438	332	150	69
Senior male	1239	315	275	231	203	144	53	18
Senior female	1483	340	314	258	235	188	97	51
Ratio male/female	0.84	0.93	0.88	0.90	0.86	0.77	0.55	0.35
Ratio female/male	1.2	1.1	1.1	1.2	1.2	1.3	1.8	2.8

Table 35
Disequilibrium in Sexually Available Partners *

	Total	55-59	60-64	65-69	70-74	75-79	80-84	85+
Repartition by age	1093	211	232	179	194	159	82	36
Senior male	257	19	28	45	63	66	26	10
Senior female	836	192	204	134	131	93	56	26
Ratio male/female	0.31	0.10	0.14	0.34	0.48	0.71	0.46	0.38
Ratio female/male	3.25	10.1	7.29	3.0	2.1	1.4	2.2	2.6

* In this table, no difference is made between sexually inactive and sexually deprived. They are both considered as sexually available, i.e. without spouse or permanent companion.

Table 36

Love, Intimacy, Attachment to a Specific Partner (N = 1070)

	Male	%	Female	%
Total seniors in love	405		665	
Love with frequent sexuality	196	48.4%	179	26.9%
Love with limited sexuality	107	26.4%	132	19.8%
Love with no sexuality	102	25.2%	354	53.2%

\# When in love, there is sex only with the loved partner, and one does not consider sex necessary for the love relationship

Table 37
Sex Without Love for Sex Partner

	Male	%	Female	%
Total sexually active population	931		471	
Total sexually active without love	628	67.5%	160	39%
With spouse	177	19%	56	11.9%
Regular companion	140	15%	88	18.7%
Outside affairs	217	23.3%	14	3%
Prostitute	194	20.8%	2	0.4%

Table 38
Sexually Active Seniors Wishing to Give Up Sex

A. Senior Male

	Total	55-59	60-64	65-69	70-74	75-79	80-84	85+
Sexually active	931	302	259	169	97	72	24	8
Wishing to give up sex	48	12	12	9	0	11	2	2
% wishing to give up sex	5.2%	4.0%	4.6%	5.3%	0%	15.3%	8.3%	25%

B. Senior Female

	Total	55-59	60-64	65-69	70-74	75-79	80-84	85+
Sexually active	471	114	96	105	68	49	28	11
Wishing to give up sex	101	28	20	21	13	10	7	2
% wishing to give up sex	21.4%	24.6%	20.8%	20%	17.6%	20.4%	25%	18.2%

Table 39
Importance of Companionship Among Sexually Active Seniors

	Male (N=931)		Female (N=471)	
Sex is more important than companionship	252	27.1%	56	11.9%
Sex is as important as companionship	306	32.9%	139	29.5%
Sex is less important than companionship	156	16.8%	228	48.4%
Hesitant	217	23.3%	48	10.2%

Table 40
Old and new sexual orgasmicity in senior women

Orgasmic before 55	203
Remained orgasmic after 55	161
Gave up orgasm after 55	42
New orgasmic	29
Masturbation before 55	66
Masturbation after 55	176

Table 41
Different Categories of Sexual Activity *

	Male	Female	Total
Category 1 (orgasmic)	721	190	911
Category 2 (masturbation)	48	176	224
Category 3 (heterosexual with poor quality)	210	281	491
Category 4 (no sex)	257	836	1093
Total	1236	1483	2719

*The three homosexual males were not included in the study

Table 42
Different Types of General Activities

	Male	Female	Total
Activity A (hyperactive)	266	212	478
Activity B (creative)	469	267	736
Activity C (moderately active)	233	285	518
Activity D (inactive)	268	719	987
Total	1236	1483	2719

Table 43
General Activity Compared to Sexuality
Male Population (N = 1236; three homosexuals not included)

Age repartition Number by age	55-59 312	60-64 275	65-69 231	70-74 203	75-79 144	80-84 53	85+ 18	Total 1236	%
Activity A or hyperactive (266 or 21.6%)									
Orgasmic (1)	87	36	39	12	6	8	1	189	71.0%
Masturbation (2)	4	2	5	4	2	0	1	18	6.8%
Non-orgasmic (3)	3	5	2	23	12	1	1	47	17.7%
No sexuality (4)	6	2	2	0	1	1	0	12	4.5%
Total hyperactive	100	45	48	39	21	10	3	266	100%
Activity B or creative (469 or 37.9%)									
Orgasmic (1)	110	110	105	28	19	11	4	396	84.4%
Masturbation (2)	4	4	6	3	1	2	0	20	4.3%
Non-orgasmic (3)	3	4	5	17	8	2	0	39	8.3%
No sexuality (4)	4	3	4	0	2	1	0	14	3.0%
Total creative	121	130	120	48	30	16	4	469	100%
Activity C or moderately active (233 or 18.9%)									
Orgasmic (1)	42	45	16	15	7	2	1	128	54.9%
Masturbation (2)	5	2	0	0	1	0	0	8	3.5%
Non-orgasmic (3)	10	9	4	21	11	1	0	56	24.0%
No sexuality (4)	7	4	11	4	8	4	3	41	17.6%
Total mod. active	64	60	31	40	27	7	4	233	100%
Activity D or inactive (268 or 21.6%)									
Orgasmic (1)	1	3	1	2	1	0	0	8	3.0%
Masturbation (2)	2	0	0	0	0	0	0	2	0.7%
Non-orgasmic (3)	22	18	2	15	10	0	0	68	25.4%
No sexuality (4)	2	19	28	59	55	20	7	190	70.9%
Total inactive	27	40	32	76	66	20	7	268	100%

Table 44
Sexuality compared to general activity
Male Population (N=1236; three homosexual not included)

Age repartition Number by age	55-59 312	60-64 275	65-69 231	70-74 203	75-79 144	80-84 53	85+ 18	Total 1236	%
(1) Orgasmic with heterosexuality (N=721 or 58.2%)									
Activity A	87	36	39	12	6	8	1	189	26.2%
Activity B	110	119	105	28	19	11	4	396	54.9%
Activity C	42	45	16	25	7	2	1	128	17.8%
Activity D	1	3	1	2	1	0	0	8	1.1%
Total Orgasmic	240	203	161	57	33	21	6	721	100%
(2) Orgasmic with masturbation (N=48 or 3.9%)									
Activity A	4	2	5	4	2	0	1	18	37.5%
Activity B	4	4	6	3	1	2	0	20	41.7%
Activity C	5	2	0	0	1	0	0	8	16.7%
Activity D	2	0	0	0	0	0	0	2	4.1$
Total Masturbation	15	8	11	7	4	2	1	48	100%
(3) Heterosexuality non-orgasm (N=210 or 17%)									
Activity A	3	5	2	23	12	1	1	47	22.4%
Activity B	3	4	5	17	8	2	0	39	18.6%
Activity C	10	9	4	21	11	1	0	56	26.6%
Activity D	22	18	3	15	10	0	0	68	32.4%
Total non-orgasmic	38	36	14	76	41	4	1	210	100%
(4) No Sexuality (N=257 or 20.8%)									
Activity A	6	2	2	0	1	1	0	12	4.7%
Activity B	4	3	4	0	2	1	0	14	5.4%
Activity C	7	4	11	4	8	4	3	41	16.0%
Activity D	2	19	28	59	55	20	7	190	73.9%
Total No sex	19	28	45	63	66	26	10	257	100%

Table 45
General activity compared to sexuality
Female population (N=1483)

Age repartition Number by age	55-59 340	60-64 314	65-69 258	70-74 235	75-79 188	80-84 97	85+ 51	Total 1483	%
Activity A or hyperactivity (N=212 or 14.3%)									
Hetero orgasm (1)	11	14	12	5	15	6	2	65	30.7%
Masturbation (2)	15	6	8	14	19	7	3	72	34.0%
Non-orgasm sex (3)	17	11	5	6	2	0	0	41	19.3%
No sexuality (4)	13	17	2	2	0	0	0	34	16.0%
Total hyperactive	56	48	27	27	36	13	5	212	100%
Activity B or creativity (N=267 or 18%)									
Hetero orgasm (1)	19	16	17	19	12	5	4	92	34.5%
Masturbation (2)	18	8	11	19	23	6	10	95	35.5%
Non-orgasm sex (3)	7	0	11	6	0	0	0	24	9.0%
No sexuality (4)	14	8	7	17	7	3	0	56	21.0%
Total creative	58	32	46	61	42	14	14	267	100%
Activity C or moderate activity (N=285 or 19.2%)									
Hetero orgasm (1)	3	3	8	4	8	0	2	28	9.8%
Masturbation (2)	1	0	0	3	3	0	0	7	2.5%
Non-orgasm sex (3)	30	28	19	10	6	1	0	94	33.0%
No sexuality (4)	59	42	20	15	14	4	2	156	54.7%
Total moderate activity	93	73	47	32	31	5	4	285	100%
Activity D or no activity (N=719 or 48.5%)									
Hetero orgasm (1)	2	3	0	0	0	0	0	5	0.7%
Masturbation (2)	0	0	0	0	1	0	1	2	0.3%
Non-orgasmic sex(3)	25	21	33	18	6	16	3	122	17.0%
No sexuality (4)	106	137	105	97	72	49	24	590	82.0%
Total inactive	133	161	138	115	79	65	28	719	100%

Table 46
Sexuality compared to general activity
Female population (N = 1483)

Repartition be age Number by age	55-59 340	60-64 314	65-69 258	70-74 235	75-79 188	80-84 97	85 + 51	Total 1483	%
(1) Orgasm with heterosexuality (N = 190 or 12.8%)									
Activity A	11	14	12	5	15	6	2	65	34.2%
Activity B	19	16	17	19	12	5	4	92	48.5%
Activity C	3	3	8	4	8	0	2	28	14.7%
Activity D	2	3	0	0	0	0	0	5	2.6%
Total orgasmic	35	36	37	28	35	11	8	190	100%
(2) Orgasmic with masturbation (N = 176 or 11.9%)									
Activity A	15	6	8	14	19	7	3	72	40.9%
Activity B	18	8	11	19	23	6	10	95	54.0%
Activity C	1	0	0	3	3	0	0	7	4.0%
Activity D	0	0	0	0	1	0	1	2	1.2%
Total masturbation	34	14	19	36	46	13	14	176	100%
(3) Non-orgasmic heterosexuality (N = 281 or 18.9%)									
Activity A	17	11	5	6	2	0	0	41	14.6%
Activity B	7	0	11	6	0	0	0	24	8.5%
Activity C	30	28	19	10	6	1	0	94	33.5%
Activity D	25	21	33	18	6	16	3	122	43.4%
Total non-orgasmic	79	60	68	40	14	17	3	281	100%
(4) No sexuality (836 or 56.4%)									
Activity A	13	17	2	2	0	0	0	34	4.0%
Activity B	14	8	7	17	7	3	0	56	6.7%
Activity C	59	42	20	15	14	4	2	156	18.7%
Activity D	106	137	105	97	72	49	24	590	70.6%
Total Non sexual	192	204	134	131	93	56	26	836	100%

Table 47
Comparing general activity before and after 55

	Men	Women
Total population	1239	1483
Inactive seniors	268	719
Active seniors	971	764
Same activity	625	250
Different activity	346	514

Table 48
Comparison of Animal and Human Sexuality

	Animals	Humans
Role of hormones	+ + + +	+
Driving force	Purely biological	Mostly cerebral (mental, emotional)
Emotion and love	0 or +	+ + + +
Individuation of partner	0 or +	+ + + (male) + + + + (female)
Posture	Mounting	Face-to-face and variations
Yearly frequency	Seasonal	All year
Awareness of pregnancy (desire or avoidance)	0	+ + + +
Conscious control of sexual activity	0 (irresponsible)	+ + + + (responsible)
Sexual attraction limited to	Genital area	Whole body
Concept of beauty	"olfactory" beauty	Visual beauty
Variety in sexual practice	0	+ + + +

FIGURES

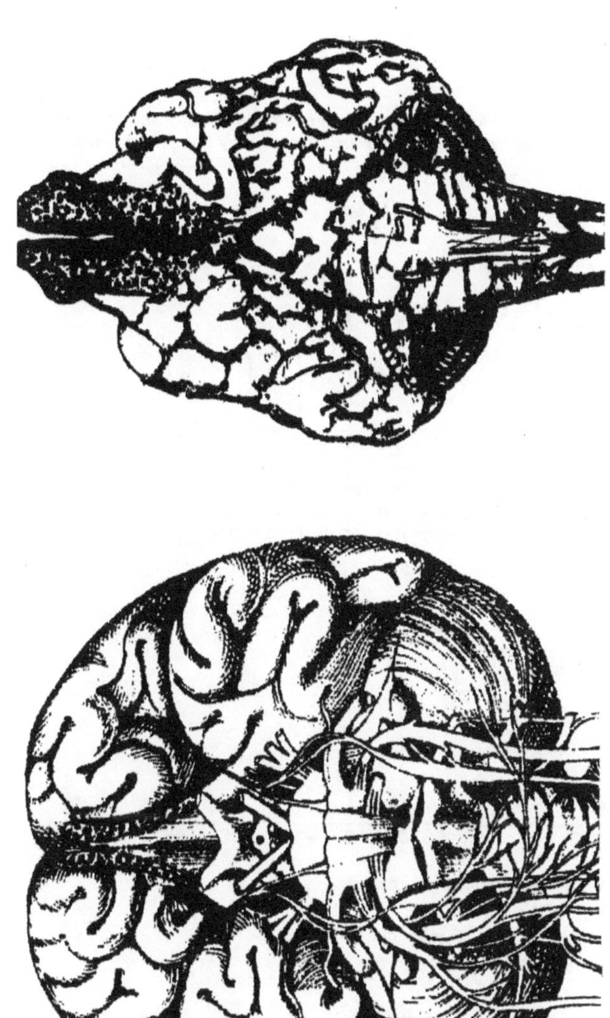

Human Brain

Upper middle zipper-like rendition shows dotted lines constituting the olfactory zone in the human brain.

Dog Brain

Right base of the brain in the dog. The same olfactory zone is much larger than in the human brain.

Difference in age between spouses (or companions) among seniors whose relationship was established well before they became seniors

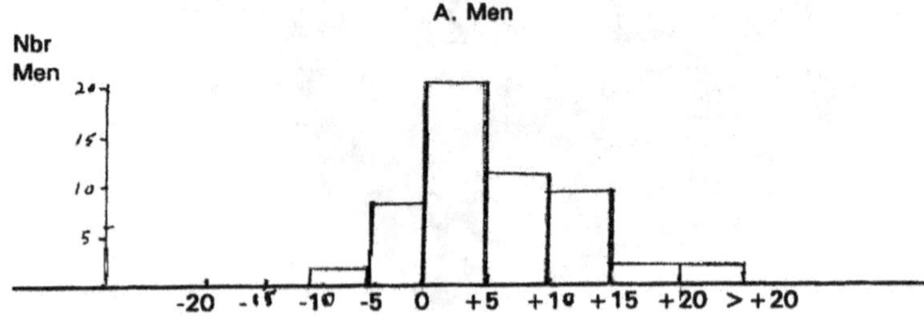

N.B. + positive means man older than woman
- negative means man younger than man
- on the average, the man is 6 years older than HIS partner

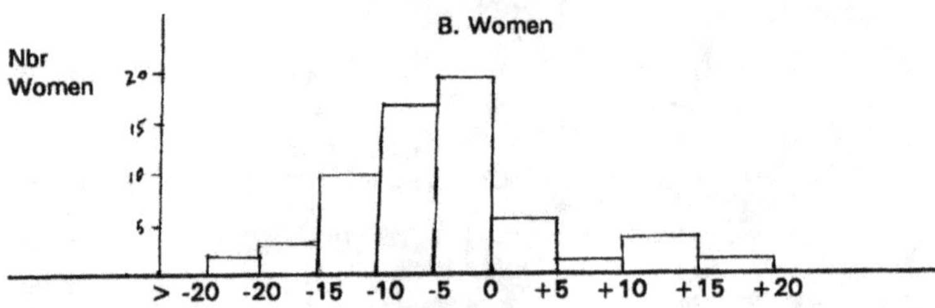

N.B. + positive means woman older than man
- negative means woman younger than man
- on the average, the woman is 5.3 years older than HER partner

Difference in age between new spouses (or companions). The relationship is established in senior age

A. Senior Men

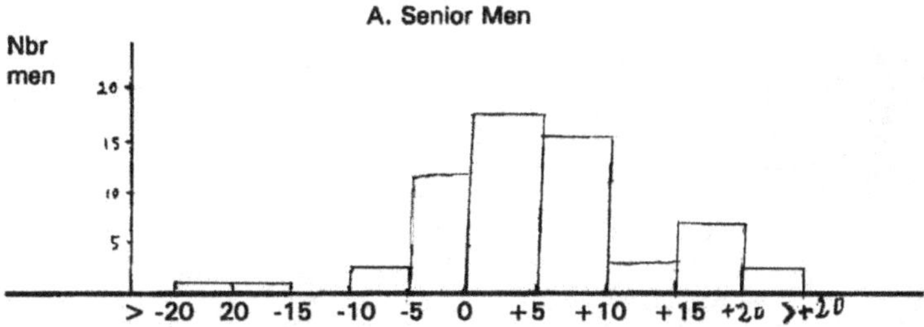

N.B. **+positive means men older than women**
- negative means men younger than women
- on the average, the senior man is 4.5 years older than HIS new partner

B. Senior Women

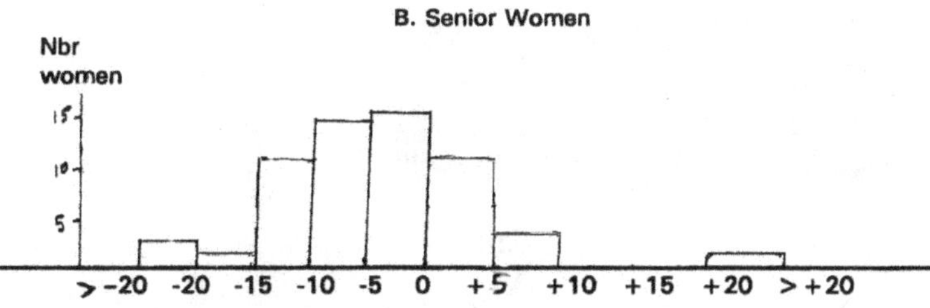

N.B. **+ positive means women older than men**
- negative means women younger than men
- on the average, the senior woman is 4.6 years younger than HER new partner

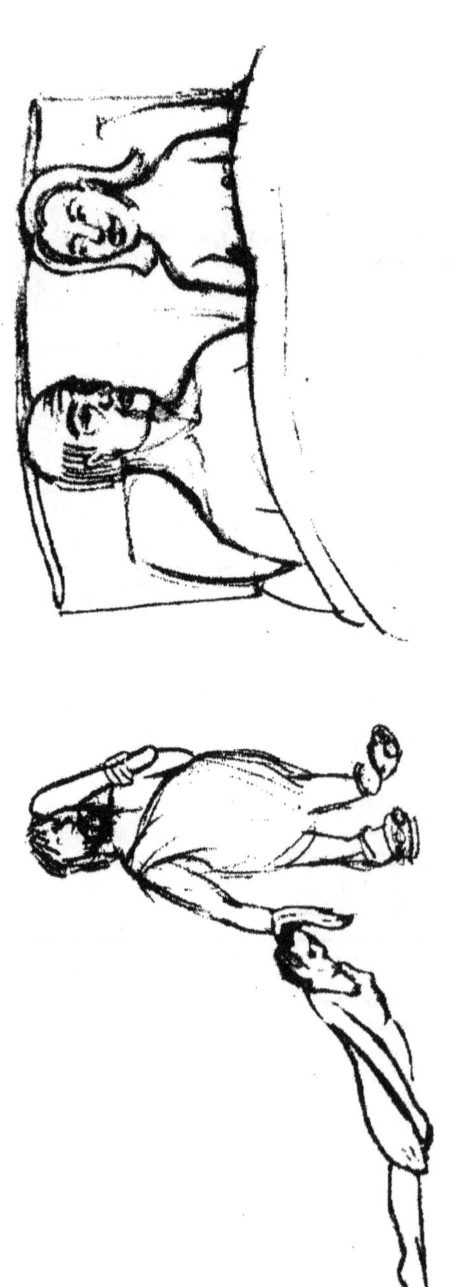

Conquest of the woman, the old fashioned way.

Sorry, grandpa. Next time we'll do better. $150, please!

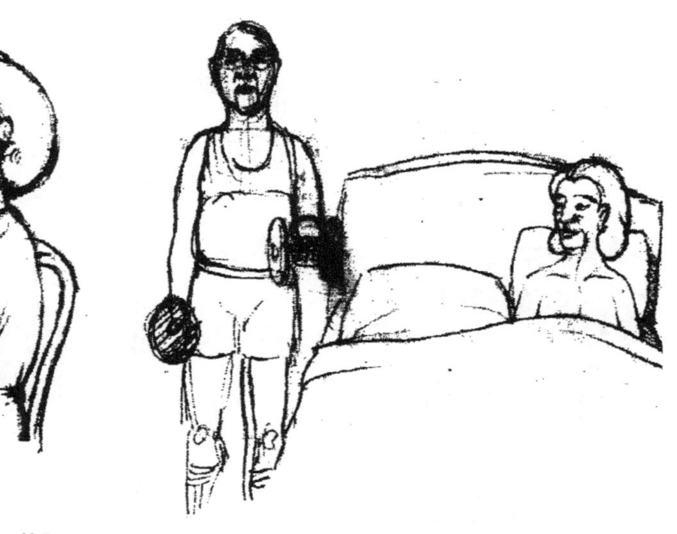

I kept looking for the perfect partner, until I finally found her. It did not work because she was also looking for the perfect partner.

Please save some of your energy for me!

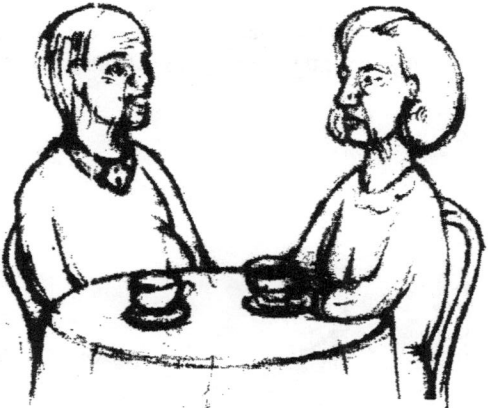

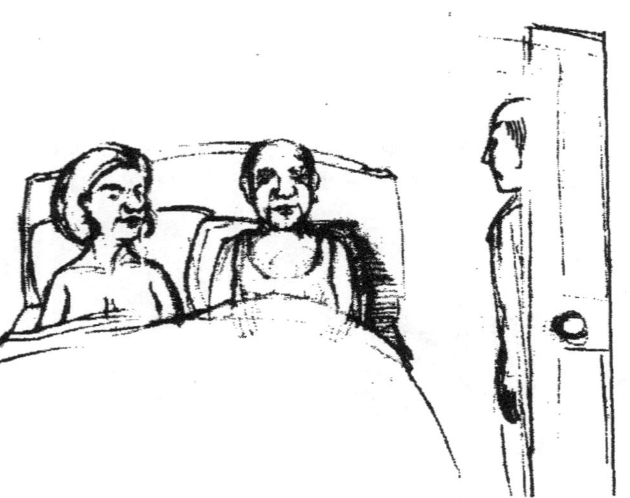

In OUR bedroom, in OUR own bed?! Couldn't you at least have done it somewhere else?!

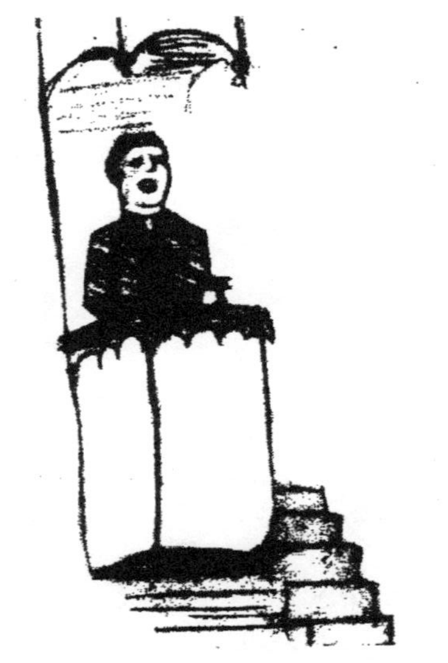

There is no sex among seniors in our community. And if there is, I hope it will never be known!

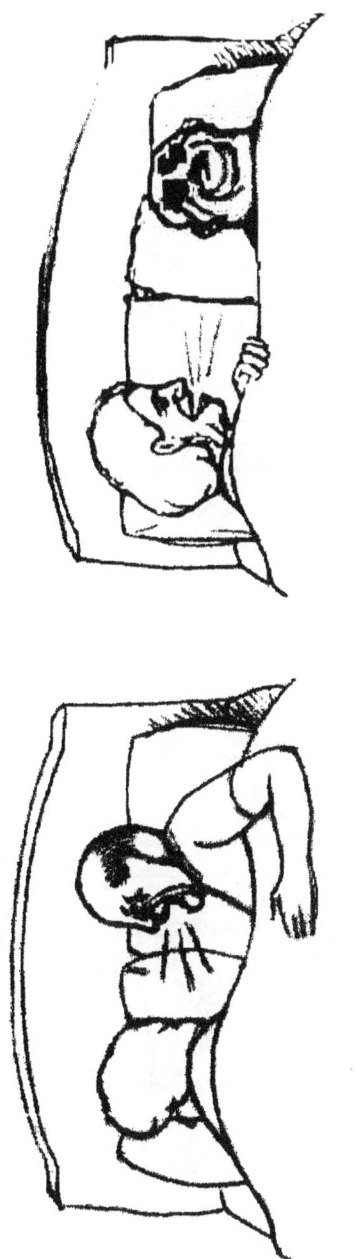

Stop turning your back to me! I know you're not sleeping....

You are not sleeping, and if you are, WAKE UP!

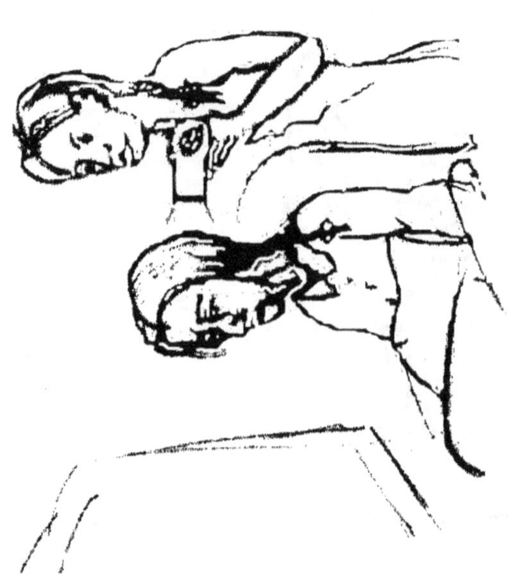

I don't like this hairstyle. It makes me look old!

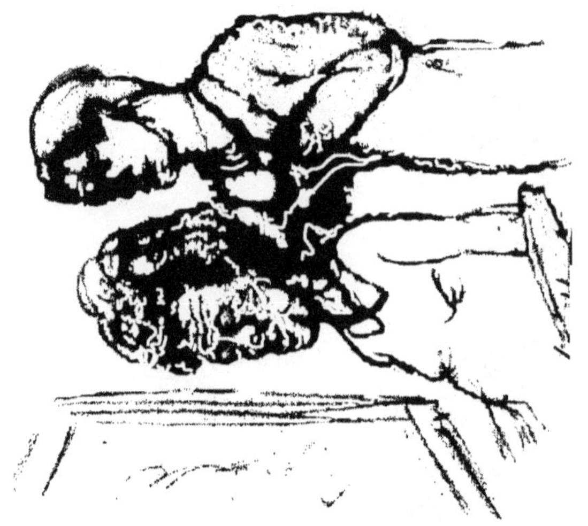

That's better!

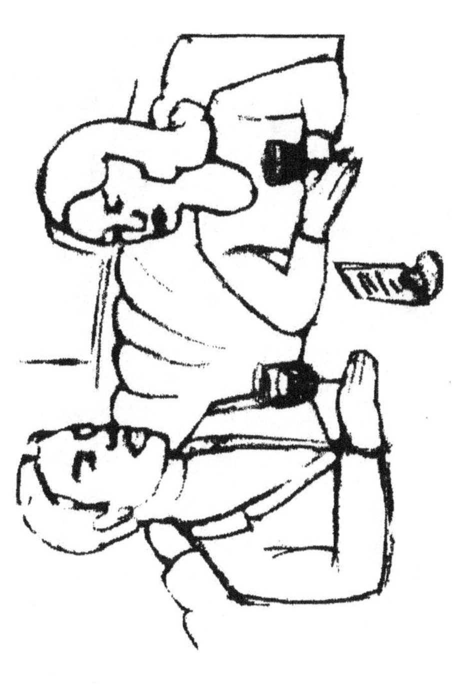

Your parents have more sex than we do? My parents do too. I tell you what: wait until we get older! I will be more potent, and you will be less frigid. Then we can have a good time!

www.ingramcontent.com/pod-product-compliance
Lightning Source LLC
Chambersburg PA
CBHW031145270326
41931CB00006B/150